I0470689

Screening for Post-Traumatic Stress Disorder (PTSD) in Primary Care: A Systematic Review

January 2013

Prepared for:
Department of Veterans Affairs
Veterans Health Administration
Quality Enhancement Research Initiative
Health Services Research & Development Service
Washington, DC 20420

Prepared by:
Evidence-based Synthesis Program (ESP) Center
Minneapolis VA Medical Center
Minneapolis, MN
Timothy J. Wilt, M.D., M.P.H., Director

Investigators:
Principal Investigator:
Michele Spoont, Ph.D.

Co-Investigators:
Paul Arbisi, Ph.D.
Steven Fu, M.D.
Nancy Greer, Ph.D.
Shannon Kehle-Forbes, Ph.D.
Laura Meis, Ph.D.

Research Associate:
Indulis Rutks, B.S.

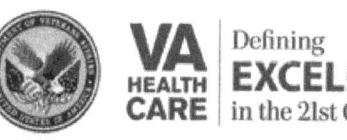

PREFACE

Quality Enhancement Research Initiative's (QUERI) Evidence-based Synthesis Program (ESP) was established to provide timely and accurate syntheses of targeted healthcare topics of particular importance to Veterans Affairs (VA) managers and policymakers, as they work to improve the health and healthcare of Veterans. The ESP disseminates these reports throughout VA.

QUERI provides funding for four ESP Centers and each Center has an active VA affiliation. The ESP Centers generate evidence syntheses on important clinical practice topics, and these reports help:

- develop clinical policies informed by evidence,
- guide the implementation of effective services to improve patient outcomes and to support VA clinical practice guidelines and performance measures, and
- set the direction for future research to address gaps in clinical knowledge.

In 2009, the ESP Coordinating Center was created to expand the capacity of QUERI Central Office and the four ESP sites by developing and maintaining program processes. In addition, the Center established a Steering Committee comprised of QUERI field-based investigators, VA Patient Care Services, Office of Quality and Performance, and Veterans Integrated Service Networks (VISN) Clinical Management Officers. The Steering Committee provides program oversight, guides strategic planning, coordinates dissemination activities, and develops collaborations with VA leadership to identify new ESP topics of importance to Veterans and the VA healthcare system.

Comments on this evidence report are welcome and can be sent to Nicole Floyd, ESP Coordinating Center Program Manager, at nicole.floyd@va.gov.

Recommended citation: Spoont M, Arbisi P, Fu S, Greer N, Kehle-Forbes S, Meis L, Rutks I, Wilt TJ. Screening for Post-Traumatic Stress Disorder (PTSD) in Primary Care: A Systematic Review. VA-ESP Project #09-009; 2013.

TABLE OF CONTENTS

EXECUTIVE SUMMARY

BACKGROUND

To minimize treatment delays and to maximize population reach, Veterans Affairs (VA) established a screening program to facilitate identification of post-traumatic stress disorder (PTSD) in their patients as they present in primary care clinics. Such screening programs may be helpful because primary care providers often have difficulty identifying PTSD in their patients and PTSD is frequently undertreated in the primary care setting.[1,2] The premise of this type of screening program is to facilitate mental health treatment engagement earlier in the course of the illness and to engage patients in treatment who might otherwise not be identified as needing mental health care.[3]

Recently, the Institute of Medicine (IOM) released a report examining the screening, diagnosis, treatment, and rehabilitation services for military Veterans and service members with PTSD in the Department of Veterans Affairs and the Department of Defense.[3] As noted in the IOM report and elsewhere, successful screening programs utilize instruments that are simple, valid, precise, and acceptable both clinically and socially.[3-5] To identify screening tools that are best suited to the primary care setting, this evidence synthesis report reviews the literature on the feasibility and diagnostic accuracy of screening tools used and evaluated with a gold standard in a primary care setting.

We addressed the following key questions:

Key Question #1. What tools are used to screen for PTSD in primary care settings, and what are their characteristics (i.e., length, format/administration, response scale)?

Key Question #2. What are the psychometric properties and utility of the screening tools (sensitivity, specificity, likelihood ratios, predictive values, area under curve, reliability)?

Key Question #3. What information is there about the implementability (e.g., ease of administration, patient satisfaction) of PTSD screening tools in primary care clinics?

Key Question #4. Do the psychometric properties and utility of each of the screening tools differ according to age, gender, race/ethnicity, substance abuse, or other comorbidities?

METHODS

We searched Ovid MEDLINE from 1981 to October 2012 using standard search terms (Appendix A). We limited the search to peer-reviewed articles involving human subjects and published in the English language. We also searched the National Center for PTSD's Published International Literature On Traumatic Stress (PILOTS) database (http://www.ptsd.va.gov/professional/pilots-database/pilots-assessment.asp). A similar search strategy was used (Appendix A). Additional citations were identified from reference lists of relevant articles and existing reviews.

Titles, abstracts, and articles were reviewed by researchers trained in the critical analysis of literature. We excluded studies that did not involve screening of adults in primary care settings in the United States, that did not report an evaluation of a tool for screening for PTSD, that did not include a gold-standard assessment of PTSD as a comparator, and that did not report outcomes of interest (diagnostic accuracy or information related to implementation of a screening tool). Qualifying gold-standard interviews used in the included studies are presented in Table 1.

Study characteristics, patient characteristics, and outcomes were extracted by co-investigators under the supervision of the Principal Investigator, a VA psychologist and core investigator. We assessed study quality based on selected criteria from the QUality Assessment of Studies of Diagnostic Accuracy included in Systematic reviews (QUADAS) tool.[6] We determined levels of evidence according to the system developed for the Rational Clinical Examination series.[7] Findings were narratively summarized.

DATA SYNTHESIS

We constructed evidence tables showing sample characteristics (screening sample and interview sample), methodological quality, gold standard (diagnostic) assessment method, and outcomes (sensitivity, specificity, positive and negative predictive values, area under receiver operating characteristic [ROC] curve, and positive and negative likelihood ratios) organized by screening instrument. We compiled a summary of findings for each question based on qualitative and semi-quantitative synthesis of the results. We identified and highlighted findings from studies involving Veterans and military personnel.

PEER REVIEW

A draft version of this report was reviewed by technical experts, as well as clinical leadership. Reviewer comments were addressed and our responses incorporated in the final report (Appendix D).

RESULTS

We screened 1998 titles (1302 from MEDLINE and 696 unique abstracts identified in the PILOTS database) and rejected 1844 because they did not meet inclusion criteria. We performed a more detailed review on 154 articles. With one article added from hand searching, we identified fifteen eligible studies that addressed one of the key questions.

Key Question #1. What tools are used to screen for PTSD in primary care settings, and what are their characteristics (i.e., length, format/administration, response scale)?

There were fifteen studies that used gold standard diagnostic clinical interviews to investigate twelve screening tools in primary care settings. Of those twelve tools, seven screen exclusively for PTSD and the remaining five screen for the psychiatric disorders commonly encountered and treated by primary care providers, including PTSD. Most studies had methodologic limitations including non-random screening, selective recruitment for diagnostic interviews, and diagnostic interviews conducted with knowledge of screen results. These limited the strength of the evidence base and decreased our confidence in study findings. Seven of the studies used Veteran or military samples.

Three of the screening tools also included in the review were truncated versions of longer screens. All screens were self-administered paper and pencil screening tests, and ranged from one to twenty-seven items. Response options for screen items ranged from dichotomous scoring (yes/no) to 5 point graded frequency or severity scales.

Key Question #2. What are the psychometric properties and utility of the screening tools (sensitivity, specificity, likelihood ratios, predictive values, area under curve, reliability)?

Few studies examining the use of PTSD screening tools in primary care settings were of high quality, and only one was conducted in VA.[8] The Primary Care-PTSD (PC-PTSD), which is the screen currently used in VA, was evaluated in three studies all of moderate methodologic quality.[9-11] In the initial derivative study, the PC-PTSD had a sensitivity of 77% and a specificity of 85%, yielding positive and negative likelihood ratios of 5.1 and 0.27 respectively at the recommended cut-off. Across the three studies, positive likelihood ratios ranged from 3.6 to 5.1, and negative likelihood ratios were less than 0.30.

The most commonly used screening tools (PC-PTSD, SPAN [**S**tartle, **P**hysiological arousal to reminders, **A**nger, and **N**umbness], PTSD Checklist, Breslau Scale) demonstrated reasonable performance characteristics with positive likelihood ratios generally ranging from 3.0 to 10.0 and negative likelihood ratios between 0.20 to 0.42. Very short screens (i.e., one or two items) performed less well, with positive likelihood ratios less than 3.0, making them less clinically useful.

The determination of optimal cut scores depends on the prevalence of PTSD in the target population, and whether the primary intent of the screen is to maximize identification of possible patients with PTSD (i.e., sensitivity) or to more precisely deploy limited clinical resources to follow-up positive screens (i.e., maximize specificity). The optimal cut-score for the most commonly used screen, the PTSD Checklist (PCL), varied across clinical settings according to differences in PTSD prevalence rates and sample compositions. Because the 17 item screen has a more graded scoring distribution, optimal cut-scores could be more precisely determined for a given clinical setting. In contrast, across studies, the intermediate length screens all had sharp drop-offs just under the recommended cut-scores. This suggests that the optimal cut score of an intermediate length screen is less likely to vary across populations and settings, and can therefore be more easily adopted by different healthcare systems. However, it also means that there is a steeper trade-off between sensitivity and specificity in cut-scores that differ only by one point, which may have significant policy and resource implications.

Key Question #3. What information is there about the implementability (e.g., ease of administration, patient satisfaction) of PTSD screening tools in primary care clinics?

Although most screens were constructed with brevity and ease of administration in mind, only three studies[12-14] examined the time it took for patients to complete the screening tools and only one of these[12] conducted a process evaluation to examine the impact of screen implementation on the clinical process. The longest screening tool (27 items) was reported to have an administration time of only 5-10 minutes to complete, suggesting that none of the screens posed a significant time burden on patients. In the one study that conducted an implementation evaluation, both patients and providers found use of the screening tool helpful and acceptable, and that it facilitated discussion of mental health issues in the clinical encounter.

Key Question #4. Do the psychometric properties and utility of each of the screening tools differ according to age, gender, race/ethnicity, substance abuse, or other comorbidities?

There is very little information about screen performance characteristics across demographic and diagnostic groups. There were two studies that examined differential performance characteristics of the screening tool used by VA (PC-PTSD) and in both there was weak evidence that the PC-PTSD performs less well for women than for men. The reason for this is currently unknown. High quality studies are needed to determine if PTSD in women is missed using the cut-score currently employed in clinical settings.

There is also weak evidence that the PCL performs less well for younger African American Veterans, although performance characteristics are still in the acceptable range. More research would be needed to determine whether use of the PCL in clinical settings leads to race disparities among younger African American Veterans.

Although psychiatric comorbidity among Veterans with PTSD is common, there is no information about the impact of specific psychiatric conditions (e.g., traumatic brain injury) on the performance characteristics of any of the screening tools as administered in the primary care setting.

FUTURE RESEARCH

1. The new Diagnostic Statistical Manual-5 (DSM-5) diagnostic criteria for PTSD are soon to be released. Although it is unlikely that the overall performance of the screening tool used by VA (PC-PTSD) and other tools reviewed in this report will be appreciably altered given the new diagnostic criteria, the importance of PTSD detection and treatment in VA requires a high degree of confidence in tools used in clinical care of Veterans with PTSD. Accordingly, the PC-PTSD should be validated against the DSM-5 PTSD criteria.

2. VA has worked to minimize healthcare disparities. Because there is weak and inconsistent evidence of possible variation in screen performance related to patient characteristics, more information is needed to determine whether screening tools for PTSD work equally well regardless of patient age, gender, race, ethnicity.

3. Although psychiatric comorbidity is common among Veterans with PTSD, there is no information about whether the performance of screening tools is altered in the presence of specific psychiatric comorbidities as they present in primary care clinics.

4. There are no studies examining the impact of mental health screening on the primary care encounter within the VA system, and only one implementation study was done in a

community setting. It would be helpful to have more information about how PTSD screens can be best integrated into clinical practice.

5. The success of a screening program depends on whether identification of the target condition in the population improves the outcome of those who have the condition.[3,5] As noted in the IOM report,[3] this is assumed to be true for PTSD but has never been proven. It would be helpful to know the impact on the mental and physical health of the VA population, as well as the financial and opportunity costs to the VA health care system of PTSD screening implementation. To adequately address this important clinical and research gap, a randomized controlled trial or methodologically sound comparative effectiveness trial of PTSD screening of Veterans in primary care settings is needed.

EVIDENCE REPORT

INTRODUCTION

Evidence suggests that the majority of Americans will experience a traumatic event at some time during their lives and that approximately 8% will subsequently develop post-traumatic stress disorder (PTSD).[15-17] PTSD is one of the most common psychiatric sequellae of traumatic experiences and is characterized by an intense emotional reaction to the traumatic event, and followed by a persistent re-experiencing of the trauma, avoidance of things associated with the trauma, numbed emotional responsiveness, and increased arousal.[18] Rates among military Veterans returning from deployments in Iraq and Afghanistan are much higher than that found in the general population, as high as 20% by some estimates.[19] Currently, about 400,000 Veterans enrolled in VA carry a PTSD diagnosis.[20]

Those who suffer from PTSD often have diminished functioning and a poorer quality of life as evidenced by elevated rates of suicide, hospital admissions, poverty, and unemployment.[21-31] Significant medical morbidity is also common among those with PTSD[21,25,27-32] and several age-related chronic medical conditions develop earlier.[21] Moreover, people with PTSD have higher prevalence rates of problematic health behaviors, and utilize medical care at higher rates than those without PTSD.[33-35] Although there are PTSD treatments available that have demonstrated effectiveness among individuals with diagnosed PTSD,[36] many people who have PTSD may not be diagnosed and many who are diagnosed do not pursue mental health treatment. Of those who do seek treatment, prolonged delays are common.[2,37,38]

To minimize treatment delays and to maximize population reach, VA established a screening program to identify PTSD in their patients as they present in primary care clinics. Such screening programs may be helpful because primary care providers often have difficulty identifying PTSD in their patients and PTSD is therefore frequently undertreated in the primary care setting.[1,2] The premise of this type of screening program is to identify individuals needing further evaluation so as to facilitate mental health treatment engagement earlier in the course of the illness and to identify patients for treatment who might not otherwise be identified as needing mental health care.[3]

Recently, the Institute of Medicine (IOM) released a report examining the screening, diagnosis, treatment, and rehabilitation services for military Veterans and service members with PTSD in the Department of Veterans Affairs and the Department of Defense.[3] As noted in the IOM report and elsewhere, successful screening programs utilize instruments that are simple, valid, precise, and acceptable both clinically and socially.[3-5] To identify screening tools that are best suited to primary care practice and to maximize relevance to the VA population, this evidence synthesis report reviews the literature on the feasibility and diagnostic accuracy of screening tools used in a primary care setting in the United States.

METHODS

TOPIC DEVELOPMENT

This project was nominated by David Simel, MD, and endorsed by the Office of Mental Health Services. The key questions and scope were refined with input from a technical expert panel.

The final key questions were:

Key Question #1. What tools are used to screen for PTSD in primary care settings, and what are their characteristics (i.e., length, format/administration, response scale)?

Key Question #2. What are the psychometric properties and utility of the screening tools (sensitivity, specificity, likelihood ratios, predictive values, area under curve, reliability)?

Key Question #3. What information is there about the implementability (e.g., ease of administration, patient satisfaction) of PTSD screening tools in primary care clinics?

Key Question #4. Do the psychometric properties and utility of each of the screening tools differ according to age, gender, race/ethnicity, substance abuse, or other comorbidities?

SEARCH STRATEGY

We searched Ovid MEDLINE from 1981 to October 2012 using standard search terms (Appendix A). The search was limited to peer-reviewed articles involving adult human subjects and published in the English language. A similar search strategy was used for searching the National Center for PTSD's Published International Literature On Traumatic Stress (PILOTS) database (http://www.ptsd.va.gov/professional/pilots-database/pilots-assessment.asp) (Appendix A). Additional citations were identified from reference lists of relevant articles and existing reviews.

STUDY SELECTION

Titles and abstracts were reviewed by researchers trained in the critical analysis of literature. We retrieved the full-text of potentially relevant articles for further review. We sought to include studies done in settings and with populations most relevant to the United States Veteran population. Therefore, we excluded the following: studies that did not involve screening of adults in primary care settings in the United States, studies that did not report an evaluation of a screening tool for PTSD symptoms, studies that did not include a gold-standard structured diagnostic clinical assessment of PTSD as a comparator, studies that did not report outcomes of interest (diagnostic accuracy or information related to implementation of a screening tool), and studies that had a screening sample size of fewer than 50 participants. Information about gold standard structured diagnostic interviews used as validation tools by included studies is presented in Table 1. There are other structured interviews that met our gold standard inclusion criteria (e.g., Diagnostic Interview Schedule or DIS) but were not utilized in studies meeting other eligibility criteria for this review and so are not included in the table.

DATA ABSTRACTION

Study characteristics, screening instrument(s) used, diagnostic measures, method of administration, base rate of PTSD, screening sample and interview sample response rates, and results (sensitivity, specificity, positive and negative predictive values, positive and negative likelihood ratios, area under curve) were extracted from each identified study by co-investigators under the supervision of the Principal Investigator, a VA psychologist and core investigator. We noted whether the study involved specific sample populations (e.g., Veterans, women, age over 60 years, etc.) and rated the study on the quality components of interest. The data extraction form is presented in Appendix B. A list of psychometric terms and how they are determined is included in Table 2.

QUALITY ASSESSMENT

We assessed the quality of studies pertaining to key questions #2 and #3 using selected criteria from the QUality Assessment of Studies of Diagnostic Accuracy included in Systematic reviews (QUADAS) tool.[6] As noted on the data extraction form (Appendix B), we focused on: 1) the representativeness of the screening and interview samples, 2) the time lag between screening and diagnostic assessments, 3) the number and selection method of screened participants who were interviewed, and 4) whether the diagnostic interviews were conducted blind to the screening results.

RATING THE BODY OF EVIDENCE

In addition to quality ratings of individual study features, we summarized the overall quality of the evidence for each study using methods developed for the *Journal of the American Medical Association* Rational Clinical Examination series.[7] One of five levels of evidence was assigned to each study based on sample size, independence and representativeness of the study samples, quality of the gold standard assessment procedure, and whether diagnostic assessments were completed blind to screening status. Definitions for each of the five levels of evidence ratings are presented in Appendix C, and our application of them to each study in Appendix F. Studies that met the lowest level of evidence (i.e., Level V) were excluded from the review. The body of evidence for each screening tool was evaluated qualitatively taking into account the strength of the current evidence base.

Table 1. Gold Standard Structured Diagnostic Interviews for Diagnosing PTSD

Gold Standard	Description	Scoring*	Administration Time
Clinician Administered PTSD Scale (CAPS)	Structured diagnostic interview of PTSD symptoms based on DSM-IV criteria. Assesses each of the 17 DSM-IV symptoms of PTSD as well as the impact of symptoms on occupational and social functioning, validity of responses, and five symptoms associated with PTSD (guilt, gaps in awareness, derealization, and depersonalization).[39]	Items scored for frequency (0 - 4) and in intensity (0 - 4). Symptom typically considered present if frequency $\geq$ 1 and intensity $\geq$ 2.	45-60 minutes
Structured Clinical Interview for DSM-IV (SCID)	Semi-structured interview that assesses major DSM-IV diagnoses. Interview is broken down into individual modules representing categories of diagnoses that can be administered individually.[40]	Each symptom is scored as present, absent, or subthreshold. The minimum number of symptoms required to meet diagnostic criteria must be coded as present.	Varies depending on modules administered and the number of disorders present. Generally, 1-2 hours.
Mini-International Neuropsychiatric Interview (MINI)	Brief structured diagnostic interview that assesses major psychiatric disorders within both DSM-IV (Axis I) and ICD-10. Items were developed by psychiatrists both within the United States and across Europe.[41]	Each symptom with the diagnosis coded as 'yes' or 'no'.	15 minutes
PTSD Symptom Scale – Interview (PSS-I)	Semi-structured interview for the 17 symptoms used to diagnose PTSD according to the DSM-IV. Assesses presence and severity symptoms related to a single identified traumatic event in the past 2 weeks, which differs from the 1 month time frame within the DSM-IV.[42] Has also been validated for symptoms in the last month.	Seventeen items each scored from 0 (not at all) to 3 (5 or more time per week/very much). Symptom considered present if it receives a score of 1 or higher.	20 minutes
Composite International Diagnostic Interview (CIDI)	Structured diagnostic interview that assesses both DSM-IV (Axis I) and ICD-10 conditions. Disorders are grouped in modules so modules of interest can be administered individually.	Yes/No response items and items with variable response options. Diagnosis based on DSM-IV or ICD-10 criteria.	Approximately 2 hours for entire diagnostic interview.

DSM = Diagnostic Statistical Manual
*If a study reported a different method of scoring a gold standard assessment, the method is reported in the text of the report.

DATA SYNTHESIS

We constructed a study characteristics table showing sample characteristics (screening and interview samples) and methodological quality. We constructed an evidence table with gold standard diagnostic assessment tools, base rate of PTSD, and outcomes (sensitivity, specificity, positive and negative predictive values, area under receiver operating characteristic (ROC) curve, and positive and negative likelihood ratios) organized by screening instrument. We compiled a summary of findings for each question based on qualitative and semi-quantitative synthesis of the results. We identified and highlighted findings from studies involving Veterans and military personnel.

PEER REVIEW

A draft version of this report was reviewed by technical experts as well as clinical leadership. Their comments and our responses are presented in Appendix D.

Table 2. Diagnostic Accuracy Terms Used in this Report

Metric	Definition	Calculation	Relation to other Metrics
Prevalence	Frequency of a disorder within a target population.	Number of true positives/total sample	Impacts the predictive values (positive, negative) of screening; if prevalence is low, PPV decreases and NPV increases.
Cut Score	Test score used to divide the target population or test sample into true positive and negative cases.	Ideal cut score typically based on desired sensitivity/specificity trade-off	Increasing the cut score typically increases specificity and decreases sensitivity.
Sensitivity	Probability that the screen will be positive when the person has the disease (true positive fraction).	True positives/(true positives + false negatives)	Sensitivity increases with higher cut scores. Higher sensitivity results in higher LR+ and lower LR–.
Specificity	Probability that the screen will be negative when the person does not have the disease (true negative fraction).	True negatives/(true negatives + false positives)	Specificity decreases with higher cut scores. Higher specificity results in lower LR– and higher LR+.
Positive Predictive Value (PPV)	Proportion of positive screens that are true positives.	True positives/(true positives + false positives)	PPV increases with higher base rates: (Sensitivity)(base rate)/[(Sensitivity)(base rate) + (1 – specificity)(1 – base rate)].
Negative Predictive Value (NPV)	Proportion of negative screens that are true negatives.	True negatives/(true negatives + false negatives)	NPV decreases with higher base rates: (Specificity)(1 – base rate)/[(specificity)(1 – base rate) + (1 – sensitivity)(base rate)].
Likelihood Ratio – Positive (LR+)	Ratio between the probability of a positive screen given the disease is present and the probability of a positive screen given the disease is not present.	True positives/false positives Or Sensitivity/(1 – specificity)	Likelihood ratio – positive: increases with increased sensitivity or increased specificity.
Likelihood Ratio – Negative (LR-)	Ratio between the probability of a negative screen given the disease is present and the probability of a negative screen given the disease is not present.	False negatives/true negatives Or (1 – sensitivity)/specificity	Likelihood ratio – negative: decreases with increased specificity or increased sensitivity.
Area Under the Curve (AUC)	Area under a ROC* curve. Measures discrimination of patients that do or do not have the disease using all possible cut scores. AUC=1.0 indicates perfect discrimination. AUC=0.5 indicates test is no better than a coin toss.	Parametric and nonparametric methods available depending on assumptions	Shows trade-off between sensitivity and specificity, not necessarily how test performs at cut score to be used in practice.

*ROC = Receiver operating characteristic; ROC curve is plot of false positives on x-axis vs. true positives on y-axis.

RESULTS

We identified fifteen articles that met our inclusion criteria. These studies evaluated twelve tools intended to be used as screening instruments to detect PTSD.

LITERATURE FLOW

We screened 1998 titles (1302 from MEDLINE and 696 unique abstracts identified in the PILOTS database) and rejected 1844 because they did not meet eligibility criteria. We performed a more detailed review on 154 articles. From these, we excluded an additional 140 articles and added 1 article from hand searching for a total of 15 studies that addressed one of the key questions. We grouped the studies by screening instrument. Figure 1 details the process.

Figure 1. Literature Flow

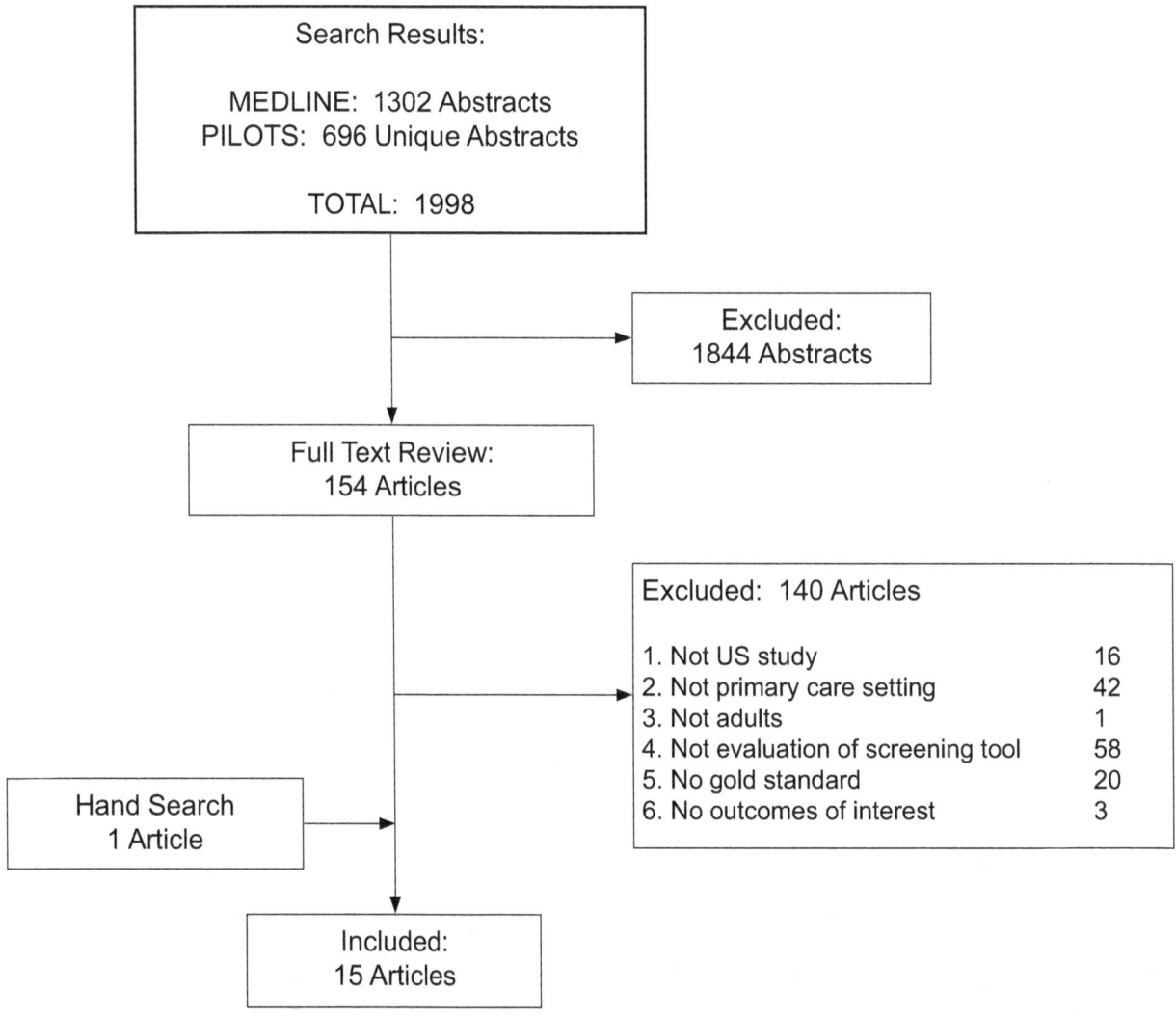

KEY QUESTION #1. What tools are used to screen for PTSD in primary care settings, and what are their characteristics (i.e., length, format/administration, response scale)?

We identified twelve screening tools that were evaluated using a gold standard structured diagnostic interview in a primary care setting. All were self-administered paper and pencil screening tests, and ranged from one to twenty-seven items. We provide a brief description of each of the screens evaluated by the included studies. The focus, length, response scale and test-retest reliability of each screen are provided in Table 3. Although the focus of this systematic review is an evaluation of the literature of screening instruments for PTSD used in primary care, we included screens for multiple psychiatric disorders or multiple anxiety disorders if there was a study that investigated the ability of the screen to identify PTSD in a primary care setting.

Breslau's Short Screening Scale

The Breslau scale was developed as a short self-report version of the National Institute of Mental Health DIS and the World Health Organization CIDI, version 2.1.[43] The initial development was done using data from the Detroit Area Survey of Trauma, a random-digit-dialing survey of 2,181 individuals, from 18 to 45 years old, living in the Detroit primary metropolitan statistical area. Respondents were asked to identify all traumatic events they had experienced and PTSD was assessed in connection with one randomly selected event from those identified. Diagnostic Statistical Manual-IV (DSM-IV) criterion symptoms of PTSD were evaluated in a structured interview and further analyses were limited to 1,830 individuals with complete data on all 17 symptoms, 142 of whom had PTSD. Items evaluating duration and impairment were not included. A model with seven symptoms (five from the "avoidance and numbing" group and 2 from the "arousal" group) was found to have higher positive predictive value and specificity than models with six or eight symptoms. In addition, a score of four or more was selected as the best overall cut point taking into consideration sensitivity (80%) and specificity (97%). In this initial derivation study, results were similar for men and women.

Primary Care PTSD Screen (PC-PTSD)

The PC-PTSD is a four item screen designed for use in primary care clinics.[9] Items are scored dichotomously as either 0 or 1 (no = 0; yes = 1). Each item was developed to map onto one of four empirically supported symptom factors proposed to underlie the construct of PTSD including 1) re-experiencing a traumatic event, 2) emotional numbing, 3) avoidance, and 4) hyperarousal.[9] Respondents are asked about symptoms experienced in the past month that were related to a traumatic event that occurred anytime in their lifetime. The instrument was designed to be appropriate for those with at least an eighth grade reading level (Flesch-Kincaid grade level = 7.7). It has a test-retest reliability of 0.83. The PC-PTSD is the instrument used within VA medical centers and community-based outpatient care clinics across the United States.

Single-item PTSD Screener (SIPS)

The Single-item PTSD Screener (SIPS) is a single item asking respondents to indicate to what degree they were recently bothered by a past traumatic experience.[10] The SIPS was developed to improve the implementation of PTSD screening in primary care clinics by providing a single, easy to memorize item. Candidate questions for the single item were written, discussed with study investigators, and then reviewed with patients to ensure the item was intuitive, clear, and acceptable. Candidate items were then refined and reviewed again by investigators before one was selected for the screen. The final selected item for the screen was, "Were you recently bothered by a past experience that caused you to believe you would be injured or killed?". Response options include *not bothered at all, bothered a little,* or *bothered a lot.*

SPAN

The SPAN is a screening tool initially developed in a psychiatry clinic for the purpose of detecting PTSD in psychiatric populations with PTSD prevalence rates around 50%.[44] The SPAN was derived from the Davidson Trauma Scale (DTS), a 17-item scale that assesses the DSM-IV PTSD criteria.[45] In order to create the SPAN, the authors split a sample of 243 participants into derivation and replication samples with the goal of identifying seven or fewer items that could be used to screen for PTSD. The result was the four-item screening tool that assesses **S**tartle, **P**hysiological arousal to reminders, **A**nger, and **N**umbness (SPAN). Estimates of PPV and NPV in a population with a 10% PTSD base rate suggested that the SPAN may also be useful in settings with a lower prevalence of PTSD, such as primary care clinics.[44]

PTSD Checklist (PCL), PCL-6, PCL-2

The PTSD Checklist (PCL) is a 17-item self-report measure designed to assess severity of PTSD symptoms.[46] Participants rate the severity of each of the DSM-IV symptoms for PTSD using a 5-point Likert scale. The DSM-IV PTSD symptoms are grouped into clusters as follows: five re-experiencing symptoms, seven numbing/avoidance symptoms, and five hyper-arousal symptoms. The PCL instructs participants to rate items in relation to stressful experiences. The measure generally exhibits good internal consistency[46] and has been demonstrated to be related to other self-report measures of PTSD as well as gold standard structured interviews for PTSD such as the CAPS. There are three versions of the PCL (original military version, PCL-M; civilian version, PCL-C; and specific version PCL-S) differentiated by the specificity of the index traumatic event used while completing the questionnaire. The PCL-M asks respondents to rate each item based on a single (unspecified) stressful military experience.[46] The PCL-C does not require the specification of a worst single traumatic event; consequently, individual symptom ratings may be based on different stressful life events. The PCL-S requires item ratings based upon a single specified traumatic experience. Several coding strategies have been applied to the PCL that can be used to indicate probable PTSD.[47,48] These include using several different cutoff scores, using DSM-IV criteria (e.g., reporting the requisite number of symptoms within each cluster at the moderate or greater level 3 or 4 on Likert scale), or using a combination of these two approaches (e.g., the requisite DSM-IV criteria are endorsed and the total score is above a specified cut point). Two short versions of the PCL were also evaluated – PCL-6 and PCL-2.[49] The two item version was created using the two items with the highest item-total correlations (i.e., items evaluating intrusive memories and distress with reminders of the trauma). The six item version was developed by using two items that correlated most highly with the total score of items within each of the three symptom clusters.

My Mood Monitor Checklist (M-3)

The My Mood Monitor checklist (M-3) is a one page, 27 item symptom screening tool for psychiatric disorders commonly found in and treated by primary care providers: PTSD, depression, bipolar disorder, and anxiety disorders (generalized anxiety disorder, panic disorder, obsessive compulsive disorder, and social anxiety disorder).[12] In addition to disorder specific symptom items, the M-3 also includes four additional questions about functional impairment. Each of the 27 questions is rated on a frequency scale from *not at all* (0) to *most of the time* (4) for a period covering the previous two weeks. The scale was constructed at a sixth grade reading level. M-3 scoring is conducted in two steps. First, the respondent must screen positive on either: 1) the suicidality item or, 2) the impairment items (any of the four items rated as *often* or more than one as *sometimes*). If either "gateway" criterion is positive, then symptom modules are scored. The PTSD screening module consists of four questions assessing re-experiencing, avoidance, numbness and startle.

Provisional Diagnostic Interview – 4 Anxiety (PDI-4A)

The Provisional Diagnostic Interview – 4 Anxiety (PDI-4A) was developed to help primary care providers quickly screen for a range of mental health disorders commonly seen in primary care: attention-deficit/hyperactivity disorder, generalized anxiety disorder, major depression, mania, panic disorder, social phobia, PTSD, obsessive-compulsive disorder, and hypochondriasis.[49] Twenty-three items from an original pool of 85 items are included in the screening tool. The instrument was developed in a sample of 343 participants recruited from 21 primary care centers. The participants were high utilizers of primary care services -- 65% of participants had 2-5 primary care visits in the past three months -- and over half reported functional disability in the same time period. The PTSD portion of the screen consists of one re-experiencing item from the DSM-IV definition of PTSD ("Having disturbing memories or dreams related to previous life-threatening events or assaults?"). If the item is rated as present at least *sometimes* over the previous week, it is scored as positive. In order for the screen to be counted as positive, however, the patient must also endorse at least one symptom listed in the screening instrument (for any disorder) reflecting in impairment in daily functioning with a frequency of at least once per week.

Anxiety and Depression Detector (ADD)

The Anxiety and Depression Detector (ADD) is a five item screening questionnaire developed to be used in primary care settings to assess possible panic disorder, PTSD, social phobia, generalized anxiety disorder, and depression.[51] The questionnaire was developed as part of the Collaborative Care for Anxiety and Panic study, and validated in university-affiliated primary care clinics in two states. The performance of candidate items (two per disorder) were evaluated on a random selection of half of their sample and then the better performing items were evaluated on the remaining half. For PTSD, the two initial items were combined into a single question (i.e., either flashbacks or nightmares). In the final screen, each disorder is assessed by a single item.

Generalized Anxiety Disorder Scales (GAD-7, GAD-2)

The GAD-7 was developed as part of the Patient Health Questionnaire (PHQ) anxiety study.[52] The study enrolled patients from 15 primary care sites in 12 states. The scale was developed in

2,149 patients and data from 591 were used to determined test-retest reliability. The seven items are scored on a scale of 0 (*not at all*) to 3 (*nearly every day*), with a total score of 0 to 21. A score of five represents mild anxiety symptoms; scores of 10 and 15 represent moderate and severe anxiety, respectively. The GAD-2 consists of the first 2 items of the GAD-7. These items reflect core anxiety symptoms. The score on the GAD-2 ranges from 0 to 6. In terms of identification of specific anxiety disorders, the GAD-7 and the GAD-2 were conceptualized as "first-step" screening tools.

Summary

There were twelve screening tools, ranging in length from one to twenty-seven items, which were used to identify possible PTSD within a primary care setting. Of those twelve, seven screen exclusively for PTSD and the remaining five screen for the psychiatric disorders commonly encountered and treated by primary care providers.

Table 3. Screens Used to Identify PTSD in Primary Care Clinics

Screener	Screen Type	# Items	Response Scale	Retest Reliability*
Breslau Scale (Short Screening Scale for PTSD)	PTSD only	7	Yes/No	0.84[a]
Primary Care PTSD Screen (PC-PTSD)	PTSD only	4	Yes/No	0.83[b]
Single-item PTSD Screener (SIPS)	PTSD only	1	3-pt scale: (Not bothered, Bothered a little, Bothered a lot)	0.63[c]
Startle, Physiological Arousal, Anger, and Numbness (SPAN)	PTSD only	4	5-pt distress scale (0 = Not at all distressing to 4 = Extremely distressing)	NR
PTSD Checklist (PCL)*	PTSD only	17	5-pt degree of bothered scale (1 = Not at all to 5 = Extremely)	0.96[d]
My Mood Monitor (M-3)	Several psychiatric disorders	4 of 27 total items	5-pt frequency scale (0 = Not at all to 4 = Most of the time)	NR
Provisional Diagnostic Interview – 4 Anxiety (PDI-4A)	Several psychiatric disorders	1 item (+ 1 other symptom) of 23 total items	5-pt frequency scale: (0=Never, to 4= Very often)	NR
Anxiety and Depression Detector (ADD)	Anxiety disorders & depression	1 of 5 total items	Yes/No	NR
Generalized Anxiety Disorders -7 (GAD-7)*	Anxiety disorders	7	4-pt frequency scale: (0=Not at all to 3= Nearly every day)	0.83[e]

*Abbreviated screens (PCL-7, PCL-3, GAD-2) scored in the same manner as the primary screening tools; reliability of PCL-7, PCL-3, and GAD-2 not reported.
[a]Kimerling et al., 2006;[13] test-retest interval = approximately 1 month; internal consistency = NR
[b]Prins et al., 2003;[9] test-retest interval = 1 month; internal consistency = NR
[c]Gore et al., 2008;[10] test-retest interval = median of 13 days; internal consistency = NA (1 item)
[d]Weathers et al., 1993;[46] test-retest interval = 2 or 3 days; internal consistency = 0.97
[e]Spitzer et al., 2006;[52] test-retest interval = within 1 week; internal consistency = 0.92

KEY QUESTION #2. What are the psychometric properties and utility of the screening tools (sensitivity, specificity, likelihood ratios, predictive values, area under curve, reliability)?

In this section, we review the studies that examined each of the screening tools and provide their psychometric properties and the Level of Evidence rating in tabular form by instrument. The studies included in the review, their focus, and their Level of Evidence ratings are included in Table 4. Rationale for the Level of Evidence ratings is presented in the final column (QUADAS ratings) of the study characteristics table in Appendix E. Detailed findings are presented in Table 5. After describing the studies, we will also specifically discuss the four studies in which a comparison was made between screening instruments.

Breslau's Short Screening Scale

The utility of the Breslau scale in VA general medicine and women's health clinics was evaluated by Kimerling.[13] Excluded were those with obvious cognitive impairment, a preferred language other than English, or an invalid telephone number. The Breslau scale was completed by 92% (n=237) of patients approached in the clinics. Of those, 57% (n=134) completed the Breslau a second time and underwent a clinician interview (CAPS) approximately one month later. The interview was completed in-person by trained psychologists blinded to the Breslau scale results. Test-retest reliability of the Breslau scale was 0.84 (p<0.001). The prevalence of PTSD in the interviewed sample was 25%. Likelihood ratios for cut scores of 4 or higher, 5 or higher, and 6 or higher are presented in Table 5. Area under the ROC curve was not reported. The authors recommended a cut score of 4. At that score, sensitivity was 85% and specificity was 84%. PPV was 64%, NPV was 94%, and positive and negative likelihood ratios were 5.31 and 0.18, respectively. The authors noted that the sensitivity and specificity were acceptable for cut scores of 4, 5, and 6. Based on likelihood ratios, the authors suggested that patients with scores of 6 or 7 should be targeted first for additional assessment.

Table 4. Characteristics of Included Studies with Level of Evidence Rating

Study	Screens	Gold Standard	Women Only Sample	Military/ Veterans	Screening Sample n (Response Rate %)	Interview Sample n (Response Rate %)	Level of Evidence Rating[#]
Andrykowski, 1998[47]	PCL-C	SCID NP PTSD Module	X		84 (79%)	82 (77%)	IV
Dobie, 2002[53]	PCL-C	CAPS	X	X	282 (11%)*	282 (11%)	III
Freedy, 2010[11]	SPAN, Breslau, PC-PTSD, PCL-C	CAPS			411 (53% eligible, 79% contacted)	Same	IV
Gaynes, 2010[12]	M-3	MINI			723 (54%)	647*	I
Gore, 2008[10]	SIPS, PC-PTSD	PSS-I		X	SIP: 3234 (est. 88%) PC-PTSD/PCL: 213 (NR)	213*	III
Houston, 2011[50]	PDI-4A	SCID			343‡	‡	IV
Kimerling, 2006[13]	Breslau	CAPS		X	258 (convenience sample)	134 (57%)	III
Kroenke, 2007[14]	GAD-7	SCID			965* (randomly selected from 92% of those invited who completed questionnaire)	965* (randomly selected from 1654 who agreed)	I
Lang, 2003[54]	PCL-C	CIDI	X	X	221 (56%)	49 (randomly selected from 192 [87%] who agreed)	II
Lang, 2005[49]	PCL-C	CIDI		X (partial)^	275 (65%)	154 (randomly selected from 401 enrolled)	II
Means-Christensen, 2006[51]	ADD	CIDI			7,738 (61%)	569 (38% +screens) 232 (21% eligible −screens)	IV
Meltzer-Brody, 2004[55]	SPAN	MINI	X		292 (76%)	32 (36%) with trauma	III
Prins, 2003[9]	PC-PTSD PCL-S	CAPS		X	335 (convenience sample)	167 (50%)	III
Walker, 2002[56]	PCL (version not specified)	CAPS	X		1,225 (62%)	152 (74%) with trauma 116 (75%) no trauma	III
Yeager, 2007[8]	SPAN, PCL (version not specified)	CAPS	Sample 2 women only	X	Sample 1: 888 (74%) Sample 2: 191 (69%)	728 (82%) 130 (68%)	I

#Level of Evidence Ratings range from I = high quality to IV = marginal quality (see Appendix C)
*Only reported on those who completed both PTSD screen and diagnostic interview
‡ Multi-stage screening, with 898 screened with self-report instrument, 704 further screened by primary care provider, 440 additional self-report instruments, and 343 interviewed.
^Results not separated for Veterans/non-Veterans

Individuals from a family practice clinic were the focus of a second study.[11] In addition to the Breslau scale, participants in this study completed the PCL-C, the PC-PTSD, and the SPAN. The study included a convenience sample of patients 18 years and older and excluded those who did not speak English, had gross cognitive impairment, or were medically unstable. Participants were asked to rate the presence of PTSD symptoms in the previous month. Screening and diagnostic interviews were completed on 411 patients (53% of those who originally consented or 79% of those contacted). The telephone interviews were conducted by experienced survey research personnel rather than mental health professionals. The order of administration of the four screening measures was randomized. The diagnostic interview (referred to as CAPS-modified because the interviewers were not mental health professionals) followed the four screening measures. Blinding was not reported but the screening and diagnostic interviews were completed in one telephone session. The gender and race distributions of study participants were significantly different from those in the clinic population. Specifically, there were fewer men, more whites, and fewer African American or other race individuals in the study population. The prevalence of PTSD in the sample was 32%. The overall diagnostic efficiency (area under the ROC curve) for the Breslau scale was 0.88. It was noted that diagnostic efficiency was significantly better for men than women. The optimal cut score was reported to be 4. At that cut score, sensitivity was 85%, specificity was 76%, PPV was 31%, NPV was 98%, positive likelihood ratio was 3.58 and negative likelihood ratio was 0.20.

Primary Care PTSD Screen (PC-PTSD)

Three studies that met criteria for the present review evaluated the PC-PTSD.[9-11] In two of the studies, the gold standard was the CAPS;[9,11] in the third study, the gold standard was the PSS-I.[10]

In the initial psychometric paper, Veterans attending general medical or women's health clinics were recruited.[9] Those with gross cognitive impairment or a primary language other than English were excluded. The proportion of all eligible patients represented by those who participated in the study or the number of patients who were approached, but declined to participate were not reported. From a convenience sample of 335, 167 (50%) completed the PC-PTSD. The base rate of PTSD was 26% based on results from the CAPS administered by trained psychologists within one month of the screening tests and blinded to the screening results. At a cut score of 3, sensitivity was 77%, specificity was 85%, PPV was 63%, NPV was 91%, positive likelihood ratio was 5.13, and negative likelihood ratio was 0.27. Area under the ROC curve was not reported.

Freedy et al. observed a PTSD base rate of 32%.[11] Details of this study are reported above. Area under the ROC curve for the PC-PTSD was 0.92. At a cut score of 3, sensitivity was 85%, specificity was 82%, PPV and NPV were 38% and 98%, respectively, and positive and negative likelihood ratios were 4.72 and 0.18, respectively.

The third study recruited participants from three military health system primary care clinics.[10] Of 3,234 participants who completed the Single-item PTSD Screener (SIPS, see below) and agreed to further evaluation, a sampling procedure was developed to include a mix of individuals who responded "bothered a lot," "not bothered," and "bothered a little." Of 229 who were invited and consented to a longer assessment involving the PC-PTSD and a structured diagnostic interview (PSS-I), interviews were completed in 213 (93% of those who consented; 6.6% of those who were initially screened). The PSS-I was administered by trained mental health professionals blinded to the SIPS results. Due to the sampling method, base rate could not be determined but was estimated by the study authors to be 9%. Although the sampling was stratified and the sample size was moderate for this study, they used sampling weights and propensity scores to extrapolate to the larger population. A cut score of 2 or more was considered optimal yielding 91% sensitivity and 84% specificity. The PPV and NPV were 37% and 99%, respectively. The positive likelihood ratio was 2.89; negative likelihood ratio was not reported. Area under the ROC curve was 0.89.

Single-item PTSD Screener (SIPS)

Only one study met our inclusion/exclusion criteria that evaluated the SIPS.[10] This study, as described above, used sampling weights and propensity scores to extrapolate findings to the larger population. The area under the ROC curve for the SIPS was 0.77. The optimal cut point for the SIPS was "bothered a little" yielding a sensitivity and specificity of 76% and 79%, respectively. The PPV and NPV were 26% and 97% while the positive likelihood ratio was 2.28. The authors reported moderate to high correlations between the SIPS and other self-report instruments (Spearman correlations with PC-PTSD = 0.59; with PCL = 0.63). The SIPS also demonstrated adequate test-retest reliability (r = 0.63, n = 104; p < 0.001; median days between assessments = 13). The SIPS appeared to be less discriminating with a significantly lower area under the curve (0.77, 95% CI = 0.77-0.84) than the PC-PTSD (0.89, 95% CI = 0.84-0.94). As noted by Gore and colleagues, the limited range of response options for the SIPS and the fact that it is only a single item most likely underlie its lower reliability and validity.[10]

SPAN

Meltzer-Brody and colleagues examined the performance of the SPAN in an outpatient OB/GYN clinic among English-speaking women presenting for routine annual exams.[55] On an initial survey, patients were asked to indicate if they had experienced a severe trauma. The survey was completed by 76% (292/384) of patients approached. Those who reported a trauma history (n=88) were instructed to complete the SPAN and invited to participate in a diagnostic interview (the MINI). The interview was conducted in-person by a psychiatrist blinded to the SPAN results. Only 36% (32/88) of those invited to participate (11% of the 292 who completed the initial survey) completed the interview. PTSD was diagnosed in 25 of the 32 (78%). The SPAN performed well; the area under the ROC curve was 0.75. With the suggested cut point of 5 or greater, sensitivity was 72%, specificity was 71%, PPV was 90%, NPV was 42%, the positive likelihood ratio was 2.52, and the negative likelihood ratio was 0.39. However, the strength of evidence for this study is limited by the inclusion of the trauma screening question and selection of only those with a trauma history since the trauma screening question is part of the SPAN screen.

As noted above, Freedy et al. administered multiple screening tools in a family practice clinic.[11] Participants rated the intensity of the four SPAN elements over the past month. The gold standard was the CAPS-modified. The author-identified optimal cut-score was 3 yielding a sensitivity of 76%, specificity of 72%, positive predictive value of 25%, and negative predictive value of 96%. Positive and negative likelihood ratios were 2.67 and 0.34, respectively. Although 3 was identified as the optimal cut-score for both men and women, sensitivity (89% vs. 74%), specificity (78% vs. 72%), and the percent correctly classified (79% vs. 72%) were all higher for men.

In a more carefully designed study, Yeager et al. examined the use of the SPAN in VA primary care clinics.[8] The authors identified eligible participants from 229,780 Veterans who had made a primary care health care visit in a single year to one of four VA medical centers. Potential participants were randomly selected and invited to participate through a mailing. Female Veterans were oversampled by identifying all women in a single clinic and inviting participation. The gold standard evaluation was the CAPS with a focus on current and/or lifetime PTSD. The CAPS was administered over the telephone by trained clinicians within 2 months of the screening evaluation; the clinicians were blind to the SPAN results. Among the primary care patients, the screening response rate was 74% and 82% of those who completed the screening evaluation were interviewed. Among the female Veterans, the screening response rate was 69% and 68% of those were interviewed. Completers were older and more likely to be white. Preliminary examination found no differences between the 62 women recruited and the randomly selected primary care sample, so they were combined for the primary analyses. The base rate of PSTD was 11.3%. In this high quality study, the SPAN performed well. The area under the ROC curve was 0.84. At the recommended cut score of 5, sensitivity and specificity were 74% and 82%, respectively. PPV and NPV were 34% and 96%; positive and negative likelihood ratios were 4.09 and 0.32.

PTSD Checklist (PCL)

The PCL was the most widely studied instrument, and there were eight studies that investigated the validity of the PCL in a primary care setting. Five studies used the civilian version of the PCL (PLC-C),[11,47,49,53,54] one used the PCL-S,[9] and two did not specify the version used.[8,56]

Andrykowski et al. examined an interview version of the PCL-C (not paper and pencil) in 82 women at least six months (6-72 months) after treatment for breast cancer (all women were in remission).[47] PCL-C performance was assessed against the non-patient version of the SCID I PTSD module administered by doctoral-level students at the same time as the PCL-C. Interviewers were not blind to patient screening status. Of 107 women eligible for the study, 84 consented (79%) and 82 were interviewed (77%). Current PTSD was diagnosed in 6% with lifetime PTSD diagnosed in another 4%. A cut score of 50 on the PCL-C yielded a sensitivity of 60% and specificity of 99% associated with a positive predictive value of 75% and a negative predictive value of 97%. Positive and negative likelihood ratios were 60.0 and 0.40, respectively. Area under the ROC curve was not reported.

Dobic et al. examined the PCL-C in woman Veterans seen at a single VA medical center.[53] It is unclear what proportion was being treated in outpatient medical clinics as opposed to mental health clinics. Of the 2,545 women Veterans invited to participate, only 11% were included in the study and there was no information available regarding clinical characteristics of non-participants. CAPS interviews were administered by a clinician blind to the PCL-C results. Prevalence of PTSD was 36% and the area under the ROC curve was 0.86. The authors identified a cut score of 38 as optimal and found sensitivity was 79% as was specificity. PPV and NPV were 68% and 87%, respectively, while positive and negative likelihood ratios were 3.78 and 0.26.

In a similar study, Walker et al., selected a random sample of 1,963 female HMO members and mailed a questionnaire packet that included the PCL (version not specified).[56] Using a traumatic experiences screening instrument, the Childhood Trauma Questionnaire (CTQ), women who screened positive for childhood sexual trauma were identified and solicited to participate in the study. Further, a random sample of woman who fell below the screening threshold on the CTQ were also contacted and asked to participate in the study. Participants were interviewed using the CAPS within 2 months of completing the PCL. It was not reported whether the interviews were face to face or conducted by telephone or whether the interviewers were blind to the PCL results. Of the 1,225 who completed the questionnaires 21.3% were interviewed. No information was provided regarding those who were interviewed and those who were not interviewed. Further, it is impossible to determine the base rate of PTSD in the sample since women were selected for interview based on screening positive for childhood sexual trauma; in the interview sample, 10.7% were diagnosed with PTSD. The area under the ROC curve was 0.84. At the author-identified optimal cut score of 30 on the PCL, sensitivity was 82%, specificity was 76%, PPV was 28%, and NPV was 97%. Positive and negative likelihood ratios were 3.40 and 0.24, respectively.

In addition to the PC-PTSD (as noted above), men and women recruited from general medical and woman's health clinics at a VA Medical Center completed the PCL-S.[9] Data were reported for a sub-sample of 167 participants. Both the PCL-S and the CAPS were completed in person with CAPS interviewers (trained psychologists) blind to the PCL-S score. The base rate of PTSD in the sample was 26%. Using a cut score of 48 on the PCL-S, sensitivity was determined to be 84% and specificity was 90%. PPV was determined to be 62% and NPV 94%. Positive and negative likelihood ratios were 8.40 and 0.18, respectively. Area under the ROC curve was not reported.

In the first Lang et al. study, the authors examined the full PCL-C in women Veterans seeking care at a VA outpatient primary care clinic.[54] Fifty-six percent of those eligible agreed to participate; 87% of those agreed to a follow up telephone interview, and 25% were randomly chosen to be interviewed using the PTSD section of the CIDI 2.1. The interview took place less than a month after the PCL-C was administered and interviewers were blind to the PCL-C results. The randomly selected subgroup differed from the unselected group on age, race, and marital status. Moreover, the mean score of the PCL-C of those interviewed was significantly lower than the scores of those who were not interviewed. The prevalence of PTSD was 31%. The diagnostic efficiency of the PCL-C as indicated by the area under the ROC curve was 0.89. With an identified optimal cut score of 28, sensitivity and specificity were 94% and 68%, PPV and NPV were 58% and 96%, and positive and negative likelihood ratios were 2.94 and 0.09, respectively.

Abbreviated versions of the 17 item PCL-C (two items and six items) were examined by the same authors.[49] The study population consisted of primary care patients from a VA clinic or a university-affiliated clinic. Those willing to participate completed the PCL-C and returned it by mail. Approximately 50% of those who agreed to participate were randomly selected for a diagnostic interview (CIDI 2.1). The interval between administration of the PCL-C and the CIDI 2.1 was not reported; interviewers were blind to the PCL-C score. It is unclear how representative the consented participants were of the population and how effective the randomization process was. The PCL-C was completed by 275 of 401 patients enrolled (65%); both the PCL-C and CIDI 2.1 were completed by 154 patients (37% of those enrolled). Using two items from the PCL the diagnostic efficiency (area under the ROC curve) was 0.88 and nearly identical to the AUC for the six item version (0.89). The sensitivity for the 2 item version using a cut score of 4 was slightly greater than for the 6 item version using a cut score of 14 (96% versus 92%), however the specificity of the 2 item version was considerably poorer (58% versus 72%). Other values for the 2 item version were as follows: PPV 29%, NPV 99%, positive likelihood ratio 2.29, and negative likelihood ratio 0.07. Corresponding values for the 6 item version were 36%, 98%, 3.29, and 0.11.

The most methodologically sound study of the PCL in primary care settings was conducted by Yaeger et al. in 2007.[8] As described above, the authors enrolled Veterans who had made a primary care health care visit in a single year to one of four VA medical centers. As with the SPAN, the CAPS interviewers were blind to the PCL scores. The diagnostic efficiency of the PCL (version not specified) as determined by the area under the ROC curve was 0.88. At the author-identified optimal cut score of 31, the sensitivity was 81% with equal specificity. PPV and NPV were 35% and 97%, respectively, while positive and negative likelihood ratios were 4.31 and 0.23. As noted on Table 5, increasing the cut score to 50, another commonly recommended cut score, improved false positive errors, but slightly increased the false negative rate by 3% - more concerning for an instrument used for screening purposes.

The PCL-C was another of the screening instruments examined by Freedy et al.[11] As noted above, the study population included adults attending a family practice training clinic (11% of all patients approached or 53% of those consented participated in the study). The prevalence of PTSD was 32%. Overall diagnostic efficiency (area under ROC curve) was 0.93 for the PCL-C. At the author-identified optimal cut score of 43, sensitivity was 80%, specificity was 82%, PPV was 37%, NPV was 97%, positive likelihood ratio was 4.54, and negative likelihood ratio was 0.24.

In sum, with the exception of Yeager et al.,[8] studies investigating the utility of the PCL as a screen for PTSD in medical settings using structured interviews as a gold standard are generally of limited quality.

My Mood Monitor Checklist (M-3)

The initial validation study of the M-3 was published in 2010.[12] In the only, but well designed, study of the M-3, consecutive patients were approached in a university associated family medicine clinic. All were English speaking and mentally competent to consent to participate. Of those approached, 54% (n=723) agreed to participate. All who filled out the screening form were asked to be interviewed using the MINI by an experienced master's level interviewer blind to screening status. Within one month of screening, 647 were interviewed (89%). Optimal screening thresholds were determined on 80% of the initial cohort and then validated on the remaining 20%. The PTSD base rate was 6.3%. When compared with the MINI, the PTSD module (at the author-chosen cut score of 2) demonstrated a sensitivity of 88% and a specificity of 76%. The positive predictive value was 20% and the negative predictive value was 99%. Positive and negative likelihood ratios were 3.69 and 0.16, respectively. Area under the ROC curve was not reported.

Provisional Diagnostic Interview – 4 Anxiety (PDI-4A)

There was one study investigating the PDI-4A that met inclusion criteria.[50] Participants were non-psychotic individuals at a primary care clinic for a routine visit. PDI-4A results were evaluated against the SCID. Data were reported for 343 patients who completed a self-report screen and an interview by a primary care provider. The diagnostic interview (SCID) was administered by "trained raters" but whether the raters were blinded and the time interval between the PDI-4A and SCID were not reported. Only 17 (4.9%) participants within the sample met criteria for PTSD based on the SCID. Given this base rate, and with the PTSD and functioning items of the PTI-4A both rated at least "sometimes," sensitivity was 71%, specificity was 72%, positive predictive value was 12%, and negative predictive value was 98%. The positive likelihood ratio was 2.54 and the negative likelihood ratio was 0.40. Area under the ROC curve was not reported. The authors also estimated the performance of the screening instrument in a clinic with an 8.6% prevalence; the estimated positive predictive value (PPV) was 18%, compared to the 12% PPV in the study sample. The strength of evidence for the screen is limited by the purposeful selection of participants based on likelihood of meeting diagnostic criteria for disorder of interest, as well as a non-disordered control group (i.e., a non-independent sample).

Anxiety and Depression Detector (ADD)

One study that examined the ADD met our inclusion criteria.[51] Of 12,724 patients approached at university-affiliated primary care clinics, 7,738 (61%) completed the screening questionnaire, and 1,494 of the 7,738 people who participated screened positive for panic disorder, social phobia, PTSD, generalized anxiety disorder, or depression. From those who screened negative, 1,107 patients were randomly selected. Diagnostic interviews using the CIDI by telephone, were completed by 569 (38%) of those who screened positive and 232 (21%) of the randomly selected negative screen patients (31% overall). The interviews were conducted by trained CIDI interviewers who were not blind to the ADD results. Of the 801 interviewed, 18.5% were diagnosed with PTSD with a significantly higher rate among non-whites and 38% of the sample screened positive for more than one disorder (24% vs. 16% of whites, p<0.01). The sensitivity, specificity, PPV, NPV, positive likelihood ratio, and negative likelihood ratio for the one PTSD item on the questionnaire (yes/no scoring) indicating possible PTSD were 62%, 83%, 48%, 89%, 3.54, and 0.46. When a version of the questionnaire that included items related to panic disorder, social phobia, and PTSD was used to predict PTSD, the positive likelihood ratio decreased to 1.47 (Table 5). The authors noted that the PTSD screen had a higher sensitivity for whites than non-whites (86% vs. 76%, p<0.01) but found no differences based on gender or age. Diagnostic status (OR=5.41, 95% CI 3.4 to 8.6) and comorbid depression (OR=1.95, 95% CI 1.3 to 3.0) were significant predictors of screening status for PTSD.

Generalized Anxiety Disorder Scale (GAD-7, GAD-2)

There was one study designed to evaluate the ability of the GAD-7 and GAD-2 to detect anxiety disorders, including PTSD, in primary care.[14] Participants were enrolled from a research network of 15 primary care facilities in 12 states. Of the 2,149 patients whose responses were used to develop and validate the GAD-7, 1,654 (77%) agreed to a telephone diagnostic interview and 965 of those (58%) were randomly selected. Interviews were conducted blind and within 1 week of completing the screen. The interviews included the generalized anxiety disorder, social anxiety disorder, and PTSD sections of the Structured SCID. The interview sample had a slightly higher percentage of women (69% vs. 63%, p=0.003) and had a significantly higher GAD-7 score (5.7 vs. 5.1, p=0.01) than those who were not interviewed. Age, race, and education were similar in the two groups. PTSD was diagnosed in 83 patients (8.6%).

The sensitivity, specificity, and positive likelihood ratio values for the GAD-7 and GAD-2 were best for generalized anxiety disorder. However, similar values were observed for other anxiety disorders (panic disorder, social anxiety disorder, and PTSD). At a GAD-7 cut-point of 8 or greater, the sensitivity, specificity, PPV, NPV, positive likelihood ratio, and negative likelihood ratio for identifying PTSD were 76%, 75%, 22%, 97%, 3.1, and 0.32, respectively. Corresponding values for the GAD-2 were 59%, 81%, 23%, 95%, 3.1, and 0.51. Because the intent of screens such as the GAD-7 and the GAD-2 is to detect the presence of any anxiety disorder, the authors ascertained the sensitivity and specificity by comparing patients with specific anxiety diagnoses with those who had no diagnoses.[14] Despite the fact that the GAD-7 and GAD-2 yield acceptable accuracy for the identification of multiple anxiety disorders, the false positive rate would be much higher if used to detect PTSD in a clinic setting.

Screening for Post-Traumatic Stress Disorder (PTSD) in Primary Care: A Systematic Review

Table 5. Screen Performance Characteristics

Screen	Author, Year	Cut Points Used	PTSD Base rate	Sensitivity	Specificity	PPV	NPV	AUC	LR+	LR-
Breslau	Freedy 2010[11]	≥4	32.1%	85%	76%	31%	98%	0.88	3.58	0.20
		≥5		71%	88%	43%	96%		5.90	0.33
		≥6		54%	93%	49%	94%		7.51	0.50
	Kimerling 2006[13]	≥4	25%	85%	84%	64%	94%	NR	5.31	0.18
		≥5		76%	91%	74%	92%		8.44	0.26
PC-PTSD	Freedy 2010[11]	3	32.1%	85%	82%	38%	98%	0.92	4.72	0.18
	Gore 2008[10]	2	9%	91%	84%	37%	99%	0.89	2.89	NR
		3	(estimated)	70%	92%	46%	97%		3.64	NR
		4		47%	98%	71%	95%		24.9	NR
	Prins 2003[9]	3	26%	77%	85%	63%	91%	NR	5.13	0.27
		4*	25.0%	54%	93%	71%	86%		7.17	0.49
		3 (women only)		70%	85%	61%	91%		4.38	0.36
SIPS	Gore, 2008[10]	Bothered a little	9%	76%	79%	26%	97%	0.77	2.28	NR
		Bothered a lot	(estimated)	36%	96%	49%	94%		9.9	NR
SPAN	Freedy 2010[11]	3	32.1%	76%	72%	25%	96%	0.84	2.67	0.34
		4		53%	85%	31%	93%		3.52	0.56
	Meltzer-Brody 2004[55]	3	Unclear	80%	29%	80%	28%	0.75	1.12	0.70
		4		76%	43%	83%	33%		1.33	0.56
		5		72%	71%	90%	42%		2.52	0.39
	Yeager 2007[8]	3	11.3%	77%	73%	27%	96%	0.84	2.87	0.32
		4		75%	78%	30%	96%		3.41	0.32
		5		74%	82%	34%	96%		4.09	0.32

Screen	Author, Year	Cut Points Used	PTSD Base rate	Sensitivity	Specificity	PPV	NPV	AUC	LR+	LR-
PCL	Andrykowski 1998[47] PCL-C	30	Current PTSD: 6%	100%	83%	24%	100%	NR	5.88	0.00
		40		60%	93%	33%	97%		8.57	0.43
		50	Lifetime subsyndromal PTSD: 9%	60%	99%	75%	97%		60.0	0.40
		DSM-IV Symptom cluster		60%	97%	60%	97%		20.0	0.41
	Dobie 2002[53] PCL-C	38	36%	79%	79%	68%	87%	0.86	3.78	0.26
		44		68%	86%	73%	83%		4.69	0.38
		50		58%	92%	79%	80%		7.54	0.45
	Freedy 2010[11] PCL-C	43	32.1%	80%	82%	37%	97%	0.93	4.54	0.24
		46		75%	88%	44%	96%		6.11	0.29
	Lang 2005[49] PCL-C	2 item	16%	96%	58%	29%	99%	0.88	2.29	0.07
		6 item		92%	72%	36%	98%	0.89	3.29	0.11
		17 item – 30		96%	59%	30%	99%	0.90	2.34	0.07
		17 item – 50		54%	94%	62%	92%	0.90	9.00	0.49
	Lang 2003[53] PCL-C	28	31%	94%	68%	58%	96%	0.89	2.94	0.09
		30		78%	71%	55%	86%		2.69	0.31
		40		61%	94%	80%	82%		10.17	0.41
		50		39%	94%	75%	22%		6.50	0.65
	Prins, 2003[9] PCL-S version	48	26%	84%	90%	62%	94%	NR	8.40	0.18
	Walker 2002[56] version not specified	30	NA	82%	76%	28%	97%	0.84	3.40	0.24
		45		36%	95%	43%	93%		6.59	0.68
		50		21%	98%	50%	91%		8.57	0.81
	Yeager 2007[8] version not specified	31	11.3%	81%	81%	35%	97%	0.88	4.31	0.23
		44		63%	91%	47%	95%		7.02	0.41
		50		53%	95%	57%	94%		10.32	0.50

Screening for Post-Traumatic Stress Disorder (PTSD) in Primary Care: A Systematic Review

Screen	Author, Year	Cut Points Used	PTSD Base rate	Sensitivity	Specificity	PPV	NPV	AUC	LR+	LR-
M-3	Gaynes 2010[12]	2	6.3% PTSD 35% any disorder	88%	76%	20%	99%	NR	3.69	0.16
PDI-4A	Houston 2011[50]	PTSD item and functioning item both rated at least *sometimes*	4.9%	71%	72%	12%	98%	NR	2.54	0.40
ADD	Means-Christensen 2006[51]	PTSD item only (Yes/No) 3 items (1 specific to PTSD)	18.5%	62%	83%	48%	89%	NR	3.54	0.46
			18.5%	96%	35%	27%	97%		1.47	0.11
GAD-7	Kroenke 2007[14]	GAD-7 ≥8	8.6%	76%	75%	22%	97%	0.83	3.1	0.32
		GAD-2 ≥3		59%	81%	23%	95%	0.80	3.1	0.51

PPV = positive predictive value; NPV = negative predictive value; AUC = area under ROC curve; LR+ = positive likelihood ratio; LR- = negative likelihood ratio; NA = not applicable; NR = not reported

*Based on data from n=188 who completed the PC-PTSD; base rate in that group was 24.5%

Comparative Studies

There were four studies that compared screening instruments for PTSD (Table 6).[8-11] Two of the studies, were given Level III evidence ratings.[9,10] Although both Freedy et al.[11] and Yeager et al.[8] compared the SPAN and PCL within their studies, one study only reported SPAN statistics up to a cut score of 4,[11] which was not the optimal score in the second study.[8] Nonetheless, the SPAN performed similarly in those two studies at that cut score despite differences in the study designs. In both studies, the PCL slightly outperformed the other instruments as evidenced by higher AUC statistics; however, the difference was likely not clinically meaningful.

The PCL-S and PC-PTSD comparison in the Prins et al. study is limited by the use of a small convenience sample.[9] The PCL-S outperformed the PC-PTSD as might be expected by a longer screening tool; however, the PC-PTSD was found to have good clinical utility with a positive likelihood ratio of 5.13 and a negative ratio of 0.27.

The focus of the Gore et al. study was to identify a single item screening question that could be used by primary care providers as the first stage in a multi-step assessment process.[10] Although both the PC-PTSD and PCL-C were given to the interview sample, the PCL-C was used for validation purposes only and no statistical comparisons of the single item screen to the PCL-C were made. As would be expected, the performance of the four item PC-PTSD was better than that of the single item SIP.

Summary

Although there is limited information regarding the implementation of PTSD screens in primary care settings, what information does exist suggests that such screening can be done efficiently and that it can have a positive impact on the clinical process and is acceptable to both patients and providers. Six of the studies employed samples of Veterans or military personnel, and all of these were evaluating PTSD-specific screening tools. Screening tools functioned in a clinically useful fashion per likelihood ratio statistics in both Veteran and community samples. However, no study included both sample types, so there is no information as to whether a particular screen is better able to detect PTSD in a Veteran or a community sample. Screen length, at least up to 27 items, can be readily administered in most clinical settings prior to patients' appointments.

As can be seen in Table 4, only three of the fifteen studies were methodologically rigorous enough to warrant Level I ratings (i.e., they had independent, blind comparison of sign or symptom results with a "gold standard" of anatomy, physiology, diagnosis, or prognosis among a large number of consecutive patients suspected of having the target condition). Two, from the same investigator, met criteria for a Level II rating. Four were rated Level IV due to lack of independence of diagnostic interviewers (i.e., not blind to screening status), selective sampling of interviewees or both. Studies with Level IV ratings often overestimate the performance of the screens they aim to evaluate, thereby limiting our confidence in the strength of their findings.

Performance of the very brief screening tools for PTSD (those of one or two items) had the least discriminative power and had steep trade-offs in sensitivity and specificity between their limited response options resulting in no clear optimal cut score. Comparisons of the intermediate length screens were limited by the lack of comparative studies of sufficient rigor. Only one study directly compared intermediate length screens and that study suffered from uncorrected sampling bias and interviews not blind to screen outcomes.

Of the intermediate screens, the PCL-6 item had the smallest evidence base, and was evaluated in only one study, which limits the generalizability of those findings. Across studies, there is weak evidence that the clinical utility of the Breslau scale and PC-PTSD are likely comparable, and some indication that both the Breslau scale and the PC-PTSD discriminate better than the SPAN. However, direct comparisons of these scales in a rigorously controlled study would be necessary to increase confidence in these findings.

The PCL is the most widely studied of the screens, although only one study had sufficient rigor to warrant a Level of Evidence rating of I[8] and two studies by the same author were rated as Level II.[49,54] Across studies, using 50 as a cut score was associated with negative likelihood ratios of 0.5 or greater, indicating that the post-screen odds of not having PTSD given a negative screen were no better than what might be assumed given population prevalence rates. That is, there would a significant risk of false negative rates, indicating that this often used cut-score is too high even for a Veteran population.

The optimal cut-score for the most commonly used screen, the PTSD Checklist (PCL), varied across clinical settings according to differences in PTSD prevalence rates and sample compositions. Because the 17 item screen has a more graded scoring distribution, optimal cut-scores could be more precisely determined for a given clinical setting. In contrast, across studies, the intermediate length screens all had sharp drop-offs just under the recommended cut-scores. This suggests that the optimal cut score of an intermediate length screen is less likely to vary across populations and settings, and can therefore be more easily adopted by different healthcare systems. However, it also means that there is a steeper trade-off between sensitivity and specificity in cut-scores that differ only by one point, which may have significant policy and resource implications.

We also examined the performance of five scales that screened for multiple conditions, including PTSD (ADD, PDI-4A, M-3, GAD-7, GAD-2). None of these more general screens were assessed in Veteran samples. Of the general screens, only the M-3, GAD-7, and GAD-2 were evaluated with sufficient rigor to evaluate their potential utility to screen for PTSD. The GAD-7 was superior to the GAD-2 in terms of its accuracy in detecting PTSD among primary care patients.[14] The likelihood ratios for the detection of PTSD, both positive and negative, for the M-3 indicated that the M-3 performed better than the GAD-7 at identifying probable cases of PTSD.[12,14]

Table 6. Studies Comparing More than One Screening Instrument

Author, Year (Sample size) Level of Evidence Rating#	Screen	Cut Score	PTSD Base rate	Sensitivity	Specificity	PPV	NPV	AUC (SE or 95% CI)	LR+	LR-
Freedy, 2010[11] (n=411) IV	PC-PTSD	3	32.1%	85%	82%	38%	98%	0.92 (0.028)	4.72	0.18
	SPAN	4		53%	85%	31%	93%	0.84 (0.032)	3.52	0.34
	PCL-C	43		80%	82%	37%	97%	0.93 (0.024)	4.54	0.24
	Breslau	5		71%	88%	43%	96%	0.88 (0.029)	5.90	0.33
Gore, 2008[10]* (n=213 PC-PTSD n=3,234 SIPS) III	PC-PTSD	2	9% (estimated)	91%	84%	37%	99%	0.89	2.89	NR
	PC-PTSD	3		70%	92%	46%	97%	(0.84-0.94)	3.64	
	SIPS	a little		76%	79%	26%	97%	0.77	2.28	NR
	SIPS	a lot		36%	96%	49%	94%	(0.70-0.84)	9.90	
Prins, 2003[9] (n=188) III	PC-PTSD	3	26%	77%	85%	63%	91%	NR	5.13	0.27
	PCL-S	48		84%	90%	62%	94%	NR	8.4	0.18
Yeager, 2007[8] (n=758) I	SPAN	4	11.3%	75%	78%	30%	96%		3.41	0.32
		5		74%	82%	34%	96%	0.84 (0.023)	4.09	0.32
		6		73%	85%	39%	96%		4.91	0.32
	PCL (not specified)	31		81%	81%	35%	97%	0.88 (0.018)	4.31	0.23
		43		67%	90%	47%	96%		6.97	0.36

#Level of Evidence Ratings range from I = high quality to IV = marginal quality (see Appendix C)
NR = Not reported; PPV = positive predictive value; NPV = negative predictive value; AUC = area under ROC curve; LR+ = positive likelihood ratio; LR- = negative likelihood ratio
*Presented statistics are values adjusted for non-random sampling, therefore LR parameters cannot be directly determined.

KEY QUESTION #3. What information is there about the implementability (e.g., ease of administration, patient satisfaction) of PTSD screening tools in primary care clinics?

Although not all studies reported the time it took for patients to complete the screen that was the focus of the study, those that did indicated that briefer screens took no more than five minutes,[13] and the longest screen (27 item M-3) was reported to have taken patients only five to ten minutes to complete.[14] This suggests that none of the screens posed a significant time burden when used in a primary care setting.

Only one study conducted a process evaluation of screen implementation in their clinics.[12] Both patients and providers were administered questionnaires following the post-screening medical appointment regarding: 1) the logistical aspects of screen administration/review and 2) whether there was any change in the patient-provider interaction in the appointment immediately following screening. In terms of screen administration, only 1% of patients reported that they had insufficient time to complete the 27 item screen prior to their appointment. Of the clinicians who reviewed the screen results, 83% reported that they were able to review the results in under one minute. Most patients (70%) talked to their providers about their feelings and symptoms and 63% felt that the screening process facilitated that discussion. Of patients who were eventually diagnosed with a mental health condition, 75% felt that the screening process facilitated discussion of mental health issues with their providers. Most primary care providers (80%) reported that reviewing screen results facilitated discussion of feelings and emotional symptoms with their patients, and none found it too cumbersome.

Summary

Only three studies evaluated logistical or experiential aspects of using a screening tool in clinical practice. There was no evidence regarding readability, speed of administration, ease of interpretability, or patient satisfaction for the remainder of the instruments and no comparative studies of these implementation issues.

KEY QUESTION #4. Do the psychometric properties and utility of each of the screening tools differ according to age, gender, race/ethnicity, substance abuse, or other comorbidities?

There were six studies that evaluated whether a screening tool demonstrated demographic-dependent variation in screen validity or utility, and only four of the six studies did so systematically. All four studies that evaluated potential differences systematically examined screen performance characteristics for men vs. women. Only two examined the potential modifying effect of age or race (Table 7);[8,51] no studies examined the effect of specific psychiatric comorbidities.

Gore (2008) used demographic based propensity scores to compare the odds of PTSD diagnoses within response strata and found little evidence that demographic factors considered collectively affected screen performance; however, the authors note that with a sample of fewer than 300 people that they were insufficiently powered to adequately assess differences in screen performance between subgroups.[10] Consequently, this adds little to the evidence base regarding potential demographic differences in screen performance. Similarly, Kimerling (2006) reported that the operating characteristics (i.e., sensitivity and specificity) for men and women were "similar" for the Breslau scale, but since no comparative statistics were presented, this study was also not included in the review of evidence for Key Question #4.[13]

Of the studies that systematically examined gender differences in screen utility, findings were mixed. Freedy et al. reported that the PCL, Breslau, and PC-PTSD (but not the SPAN) were better able to detect PTSD in men than in women across all indices (Table 7).[11] Although this did not impact the optimal cut scores recommended for the Breslau scale or the PC-PTSD, they found that the optimal PCL cut score for men was different than for women (46 vs. 43). Given how close these cut scores are, it is unlikely that the utility of the PCL would differ for men vs. women in a clinical setting. More importantly, the sample used in the study was significantly different from that of the patient population from which it was drawn in that patients who were female and those who were white were more likely to participate in the study. Since no adjustments were made for this selection bias, it is unclear how this might have affected the results. Prins (2003) similarly found that the PC-PTSD was better able to detect PTSD among men vs. women Veterans, but this study also suffered from significant methodological limitations and, additionally, was based on a fairly small convenience sample.[9]

In contrast, Means-Christensen (2006) reported that the performance of the ADD was comparable for men and women, but that it was less able to discriminate cases vs. non-cases among non-whites than among whites (76% vs. 86%).[51] Unfortunately, no other statistical information was provided, and it is unclear whether this difference has meaningful clinical significance.

In the most methodologically rigorous study to examine demographic differences in screen performance, Yeager (2007) found that both the SPAN and PCL performed similarly for men as for women Veterans.[8] Although there was no primary effect of race in performance of either screen in this study, the performance of the PCL (but not the SPAN) was significantly different for white vs. African American Veterans among the younger cohort. Specifically, they examined potential race differences in AUCs for the SPAN and PCL within three age strata and found significant race differences for the PCL in the youngest ($\leq$ 49 yr) cohort, but not in the older groups (50-64 yr or 65 yr +). For those Veterans younger than 50, the PCL was a much better discriminator of PTSD among white Veterans (AUC=0.99), than among African American Veterans (AUC=0.81).

Although PTSD is associated with significant psychiatric comorbidity, there were no studies that examined whether the utility of a screening tool was affected by the presence of other mental health disorders.

Summary

There is very limited evidence regarding potential variation in the performance of screening tools by age, gender or race, and no information about how specific psychiatric comorbidities might affect the performance of the screening tools. Of the studies that were adequately powered to determine whether screen utility varied by demographic or clinical factors, only one was of high quality. Given this, our findings must be considered provisional.

There is weak evidence that the clinical utility of the PC-PTSD differs depending on patients' sex, and no information if it functions equally well among patients of different ages or racial, ethnic or socioeconomic backgrounds. For the Breslau scale the findings are similar, but were reported in only one study of limited quality. There is weak evidence that the performance of the SPAN does not vary by patient gender, age or race. The PCL appears to function comparably for men as it does for women, but there is weak evidence that Veterans who are younger than 50 and African American may not be identified as having PTSD as accurately by the PCL than Veterans who are white and/or older.

There was no information regarding the impact of psychiatric comorbidity on the performance characteristics of any of the screening tools.

Table 7. Evidence for a Moderating Effect of Demographic Factors on Screen Characteristics

Author, Year Level of Evidence Rating#	Screen	Cut Score M	Cut Score W	PTSD Base Rate	Sensitivity M	Sensitivity W	Specificity M	Specificity W	AUC M	AUC W	LR+ M	LR+ W	LR- M	LR- W
Freedy, 2010[11] IV	PC-PTSD	3	3		100%	83%	87%	83%	*		7.69	4.88	0.00	0.20
	SPAN	3	3	32.1%	89%	74%	78%	72%	No difference		4.05	2.64	0.14	0.36
	PCL-C	46	43	M: 20.0% W: 35.8%	86%	79%	95%	81%	*		17.2	4.11	0.15	0.27
	Breslau Scale	4	4		100%	83%	78%	77%	*		4.55	3.61	0.00	0.22
Means-Christenson, 2006[51] IV	ADD†			20.4% Whites: 15.5% Non-whites: 23.9% M: 19.1% W: 18.2%	NR		Whites: 86% Non-whites: 76%		NR		NR		NR	
Prins, 2003[9] III	PC-PTSD	3		24.5%^ M: 25% W: 24%	94%	70%	92%	84%	NR		11.75	4.38	0.07	0.36
Yeager, 2007[8] I	SPAN	5	6	11.3% Blacks:13.5%; Whites:10.0%	NR		NR		No gender or race differences		NR		NR	
	PCL (not specified)	31	43	M: 11.9% W: 9.1%	NR		NR		No gender or race differences		NR		NR	

M = men; W = women; LR = Likelihood Ratio; AUC = area under ROC curve; NR = Not reported
#Level of Evidence Ratings range from I = high quality to IV = marginal quality (see Appendix C)
*Gender differences found in AUC but values not reported
†Gender and age differences not reported
^Based on data from n=188

SUMMARY AND DISCUSSION

SUMMARY OF EVIDENCE BY KEY QUESTION

Key Question #1. What tools are used to screen for PTSD in primary care settings, and what are their characteristics (i.e., length, format/administration, response scale)?

Screening tools that focus on evaluating traumatic experiences are not likely to be clinically useful given the high population prevalence of traumatic events and the much lower conditional probability of developing PTSD.[3,15,38] Consequently, all screening tools reviewed in this report were those that evaluated PTSD symptoms. There is a limited number of studies examining screening tools for PTSD symptoms in primary care that examined their utility using "gold standard" structured diagnostic interviews. Most of these studies had significant methodologic limitations which limits the strength of the evidence and our confidence in these findings. Common limitations included non-random screening, selective recruitment for diagnostic interviews, and diagnostic interviews conducted with knowledge of screen results. Half of the studies used Veteran or military samples, and in these samples the following tools were evaluated: PCL (and its abbreviated versions), PC-PTSD, Breslau scale, SPAN, and SIP.

There were twelve screening tools that were used to detect PTSD, and validated using a gold standard structured diagnostic interview, in a primary care setting. Three of the screening tools were truncated versions of longer screens also included in the review. Five of the screening tools were used to screen for multiple disorders. All screens were self-administered paper and pencil screening tests, and ranged from one to twenty-seven items. Response options for screen items ranged from dichotomous scoring (yes/no) to 5 point graded frequency or severity scales.

Key Question #2. What are the psychometric properties and utility of the screening tools (sensitivity, specificity, likelihood ratios, predictive values, area under curve, reliability)?

Of the screens for which area under the curve (AUC) statistics were reported, AUCs ranged from 0.75 to 0.93. No AUC statistics were available for the PDI-4A, ADD or M-3. Performance of the moderate length screens (PC-PTSD, Breslau scale, SPAN) were comparable, though there was very weak evidence that the SPAN performed less well than the PC-PTSD or the Breslau scales. However, there were no high quality studies examining the performance of the PC-PTSD in a primary care setting.

The optimal cut-score for the most commonly used screen, the PTSD Checklist (PCL), varied across clinical settings according to differences in PTSD prevalence rates and sample compositions. Because the 17 item screen has a more graded scoring distribution, optimal cut-scores could be more precisely determined for a given clinical setting. In contrast, across studies, the intermediate length screens all had sharp drop-offs just under the recommended cut-scores. This suggests that the optimal cut score of an intermediate length screen is less likely to vary across populations and settings, and can therefore be more easily adopted by different healthcare systems. However, it also means that there is a steeper trade-off between sensitivity and specificity in cut-scores that differ only by one point, which may have significant policy and resource implications.

Screens not specific to PTSD but for which there was a study that evaluated the ability of the screen to detect PTSD performed less well than those that focused on the detection of PTSD exclusively. In some clinical settings, this might be preferable, as "false positives" on non-PTSD specific screens may reflect psychiatric symptomatology requiring further evaluation.

Key Question #3. What information is there about the implementability (e.g., ease of administration, patient satisfaction) of PTSD screening tools in primary care clinics?

Only two studies evaluated logistical or experiential aspects of using a screening tool in clinical practice. One of these evaluated the time patients took to fill out the longest screen and determined that the time investment was only between 5-10 minutes and could be completed prior to the start of the medical appointment. Only one study evaluated the impact of screen use on the process of care and found that it facilitated discussion of mental health issues with primary care providers. There was no evidence regarding readability, speed of administration, ease of interpretability, or patient satisfaction for the remainder of the instruments and no comparative studies of these implementation issues.

Only three studies reported the time it took for patients to fill out the screening instruments, and only one systematically explored patients' and providers' experiences of screening tool implementation.[12] In the study that evaluated implementation of screening, both patients and providers reported that pre-appointment mental health screening facilitated discussion of mental health issues in the subsequent primary care encounter. Most providers (80%) reported that the screen was helpful in their interactions with their patients. The authors reported that this 27 item screen of multiple psychiatric conditions common seen in primary care patients took patients only 5 minutes to complete, and that only 1% of patients felt that they had insufficient time to complete it prior to their appointment.

Key Question #4. Do the psychometric properties and utility of each of the screening tools differ according to age, gender, race/ethnicity, substance abuse, or other comorbidities?

There was very limited information regarding the modifying effect of patient demographic characteristics or clinical comorbidities on screen performance.

Of the studies that were available, there was weak evidence that the clinical utility of the PC-PTSD may be better for men vs. women, and no information as to whether its performance characteristics vary as a function of patient age, race, or ethnicity. Similarly, there is weak evidence that the performance of the SPAN does not vary by patient gender, age, or race. The PCL appears to function comparably for men as it does for women, but there is weak evidence that Veterans who are younger than 50 and African American may not be identified as having PTSD as accurately by the PCL than Veterans who are white and/or older. There was no evidence of screen performance characteristics among other minority groups. More information is needed as to whether screens, particularly the PC-PTSD, work equally well regardless of patient age, gender, race, or ethnicity so as to ensure that VA's screening program does not contribute to treatment disparities.

There was no information regarding the impact of specific psychiatric comorbidities on the performance characteristics of any of the screening tools in the primary care setting.

LIMITATIONS

There are a limited number of studies examining screening tools for PTSD in primary care that examined their utility using "gold standard" structured diagnostic interviews. Most studies had significant methodologic limitations which limits our confidence in these findings. Confidence in these findings is also somewhat limited because of variation in what studies used as a "gold standard." Although all "gold standard" interviews were based on the same diagnostic criteria, the specific interviews used, the scoring rules for the interviews, and the skill of the interviewers differed across studies. This variation may have subtly altered the performance characteristics of the screens across studies.

The appropriate balance of sensitivity and specificity of a screening tool depends on the purpose of the tool and the health care policy underlying its use. Consequently, the effectiveness of a particular screening tool depends on the precision with which the cut score is optimized given the population prevalence of the target condition and the intent of the screening program. This contextually-specific balance could not be assessed in the current review.

CLINICAL CONSIDERATIONS

Use of PTSD screening tools can improve detection of PTSD among primary care patients. While widely implemented, no randomized controlled trials evaluating the benefits and harms of screening and subsequent treatment of PTSD have been conducted. Such studies, particularly among individuals seen in primary care clinics, are needed.

The primary potential harm to the patient of screening for PTSD is the potential for misdiagnosis which could lead to labeling and potential harms of treatment. The principal harm to the health care system is that limited mental health resources become used to evaluate patients with potential PTSD diagnoses, some of whom are subsequently found not to have PTSD, leaving fewer resources available to provide treatment. On the other hand, there is also potential harm in not screening for PTSD and thereby missing cases that may benefit from detection and treatment. Not only is there a missed opportunity to treat an often debilitating illness that causes significant suffering, but there may also be a risk of allowing untreated illness to contribute to secondary medical and mental health problems. Determining the most useful instrument and the optimal cut score for that instrument would help to balance these potential harms.

Six studies used Veteran samples exclusively. Two enrolled only female Veterans. Four evaluated some version of the PCL, two evaluated the PC-PTSD, and the SIPS, Breslau scale, and SPAN were each evaluated in single studies. The evidence suggests that the PCL, PC-PTSD, Breslau scale and SPAN all perform at least as well in Veteran as in non-Veteran samples. Given the limited number of studies evaluating each screening tool and the lack of studies comparing the performance of a screen in samples with and without Veterans, there was insufficient evidence to determine whether screens were better at detecting possible PTSD among Veterans vs. non-Veterans.

Currently, the VA uses the PC-PTSD, which is short, easy to administer and has good psychometric properties. As with many shorter screens, the PC-PTSD has a steeper gradient of endorsement between cut-scores than the PCL, which may result in either an over- or under-sensitive screening tool depending on the cut-score selected and the population in which it is used. For longer screens, such as the PCL, cut-scores can be more carefully "calibrated" to the target population. However, the PCL also contains many items that may be endorsed by Veterans who have mental health concerns other than PTSD. Because of this, the specificity of the PCL is comparable to that of the more general GAD-7 when cut-scores lower than the mid-forties are used; however, use of a higher score lowers the screen's sensitivity. Whether use of the PCL rather than the PC-PTSD would improve screening accuracy is unknown.

An alternative would be a two-staged screening approach such as that used by two of the studies in the review. For example, in the study by Meltzer-Brody (2004), patients were first screened for traumatic experiences prior to receiving the SPAN.[54] However, the performance of the SPAN was not appreciably better than in other studies without the traumatic experiences inquiry. A two-stage screening approach was also used by Gaynes (2010).[12] In that study, symptom scales of the M-3 were only scored if patients endorsed either functional impairment or suicidality items. Perhaps this is the reason that the likelihood ratios for the M-3 tended to be better than those for other very short screens.

Within the coming year, the new Diagnostic Statistical Manual for mental disorders will be released (www.dsm5.org/Pages/Default.aspx). The proposed diagnostic criteria for PTSD overlap considerably with those in the currently used DSM-IV, but differ sufficiently that the performance of PTSD screening tools such as those covered in this review will need to be evaluated relative to the new criteria.

RECOMMENDATIONS FOR FUTURE RESEARCH

1. The new DSM-5 diagnostic criteria for PTSD are soon to be released. Although it is unlikely that the overall performance of the screening tool used by VA (PC-PTSD) and other tools reviewed in this report will be appreciably altered given the new diagnostic criteria, the importance of PTSD detection and treatment in VA requires a high degree of confidence in tools used in clinical care of Veterans with PTSD. Accordingly, the PC-PTSD should be validated against the DSM-5 PTSD criteria.

2. VA has worked to minimize healthcare disparities. Because there is weak and inconsistent evidence of possible variation in screen performance related to patient characteristics, more information is needed to determine whether screening tools for PTSD work equally well regardless of patient age, gender, race, ethnicity.

3. Although psychiatric comorbidity is common among Veterans with PTSD, there is no information about whether the performance of mental health screening tools, such as the PC-

PTSD, are altered in the presence of specific psychiatric comorbidities (e.g., traumatic brain injury).

4. There are no studies examining the impact of mental health screening on the primary care encounter within the VA system, and only one implementation study was done in a community setting. It would be helpful to have more information about how PTSD screens can be best be integrated into clinical practice.

5. The success of a screening program depends on whether identification of the target condition in the population improves the outcome of those who have the condition.[3,5] As noted in the IOM report,[3] this is assumed to be true for PTSD but has never been proven. It would be helpful to know if implementation of screening for PTSD has had a positive impact on the mental and physical health of the VA population, as well as the financial and opportunity costs to the VA health care system of PTSD screening implementation. To adequately address this important clinical and research gap, a randomized controlled trial or methodologically sound comparative effectiveness trial of PTSD screening of Veterans in primary care settings is needed.

REFERENCES

1. Graves RE, Freedy JR, Aigbogun NU, Lawson WB, Mellman TA, Alim TN. PTSD treatment of African American adults in primary care: the gap between current practice and evidence-based treatment guidelines. *J Natl Med Assoc.* 2011;103(7):585-93.

2. Magruder KM, Frueh BC, Knapp RG, et al. Prevalence of posttraumatic stress disorder in Veterans Affairs primary care clinics. *Gen Hosp Psychiatry.* 2005;27(3):169-79.

3. Institute of Medicine. *Treatment for posttraumatic stress disorder in military and veteran populations: Initial assessment.* Washington, DC: The National Academies Press; 2012.

4. Rona RJ, Hyams KC, Wessely S. Screening for psychological illness in military personnel. *JAMA* 2005;293(10):1257-60.

5. Gilbody S, Sheldon T, Wessely S. Should we screen for depression? *BMJ* 2006;332(7548):1027-30.

6. Whiting P, Rutjes AW, Reitsma JB, Bossuyt PM, Kleijnen J. The development of QUADAS: a tool for the quality assessment of studies of diagnostic accuracy included in systematic reviews. *BMC Med Res Methodol.* 2003;3:25.

7. Simel DL. Update: primer on precision and accuracy. In: Simel DL, Rennie D, eds. *Rational Clinical Examination: The Evidence-Based Clinical Diagnosis.* New York, NY: McGraw-Hill; 2008:9-16.

8. Yeager DE, Magruder KM, Knapp RG, Nicholas JS, Frueh BC. Performance characteristics of the posttraumatic stress disorder checklist and SPAN in Veterans Affairs primary care settings. *Gen Hosp Psychiatry.* 2007;29(4):294-301.

9. Prins A, Ouimette PC, Kimerling RE, et al. The primary care PTSD Screen (PC-PTSD): development and operating characteristics [see Corrigendum 2004;9(4):151]. *Prim Care Psychiatry.* 2003;9(1):9-14.

10. Gore KL, Engel CC, Freed MC, Liu X, Armstrong DW, 3rd. Test of a single-item posttraumatic stress disorder screener in a military primary care setting. *Gen Hosp Psychiatry.* 2008;30(5):391-7.

11. Freedy JR, Steenkamp MM, Magruder KM, et al. Post-traumatic stress disorder screening test performance in civilian primary care. *Fam Pract.* 2010;27(6):615-24.

12. Gaynes BN, DeVeaugh-Geiss J, Weir S, et al. Feasibility and diagnostic validity of the M-3 checklist: a brief, self-rated screen for depressive, bipolar, anxiety, and post-traumatic stress disorders in primary care. *Ann Fam Med.* 2010;8(2):160-9.

13. Kimerling R, Ouimette P, Prins A, et al. Brief report: Utility of a short screening scale for DSM-IV PTSD in primary care. *J Gen Intern Med.* 2006 Jan;21(1):65-67.

14.   Kroenke K, Spitzer RL, Williams JBW, Monahan PO, Lowe B. Anxiety disorders in primary care: prevalence, impairment, comorbidity, and detection. *Ann Intern Med.* 2007;146(5):317-25.

15.   Breslau N, Peterson EL, Schultz LR. A second look at prior trauma and the posttraumatic stress disorder effects of subsequent trauma: a prospective epidemiological study. *Arch Gen Psychiatry.* 2008;65(4):431-7.

16.   Kessler RC, Chiu WT, Demler O, Merikangas KR, Walters EE. Prevalence, severity, and comorbidity of 12-month DSM-IV disorders in the National Comorbidity Survey Replication. *Arch Gen Psychiatry.* 2005;62(6):617-27.

17.   Roberts AL, Gilman SE, Breslau J, Breslau N, Koenen KC. Race/ethnic differences in exposure to traumatic events, development of post-traumatic stress disorder, and treatment-seeking for post-traumatic stress disorder in the United States. *Psychol Med.* 2011;41(1):71-83.

18.   American Psychiatric Association. *Diagnostic and Statistical Manual of Mental Disorders (4th ed.).* Washington, DC; 1994.

19.   Ramchand R, Schell TL, Karney BR, Osilla KC, Burns RM, Caldarone LB. Disparate prevalence estimates of PTSD among service members who served in Iraq and Afghanistan: possible explanations. *J Trauma Stress.* 2010;23(1):59-68.

20.   Rosenheck R, Stolar M, Fontana A. Outcomes monitoring and the testing of new psychiatric treatments: work therapy in the treatment of chronic post-traumatic stress disorder. *Health Serv Res.* 2000;35(1 Pt 1):133-51.

21.   Andersen J, Wade M, Possemato K, Ouimette P. Association between posttraumatic stress disorder and primary care provider-diagnosed disease among Iraq and Afghanistan veterans. *Psychosom Med.* 2010;72(5):498-504.

22.   Breslau N. The epidemiology of trauma, PTSD, and other posttrauma disorders. *Trauma Violence Abuse.* 2009;10(3):198-210.

23.   Marshall RD, Olfson M, Hellman F, Blanco C, Guardino M, Struening EL. Comorbidity, impairment, and suicidality in subthreshold PTSD. *Am J Psychiatry.* 2001;158(9):1467-73.

24.   Smith MW, Schnurr PP, Rosenheck RA. Employment outcomes and PTSD symptom severity. *Ment Health Serv Res.* 2005;7(2):89-101.

25.   Durai UN, Chopra MP, Coakley E, et al. Exposure to trauma and posttraumatic stress disorder symptoms in older veterans attending primary care: comorbid conditions and self-rated health status. *J Am Geriatr Soc.* 2011;59(6):1087-92.

26.   Kartha A, Brower V, Saitz R, Samet JH, Keane TM, Liebschutz J. The impact of trauma exposure and post-traumatic stress disorder on healthcare utilization among primary care patients. *Med Care.* 2008;46(4):388-93.

27.   Uddin M, Aiello AE, Wildman DE, et al. Epigenetic and immune function profiles associated with posttraumatic stress disorder. *Proc Natl Acad Sci U S A.* 2010;107(20):9470-5.

28.   Schnurr PP, Green BL. *Trauma and Health: Physical Health Consequences of Exposure to Extreme Stress.* Washington, DC: American Psychological Association; 2004.

29.   Ahmadi N, Hajsadeghi F, Mirshkarlo HB, Budoff M, Yehuda R, Ebrahimi R. Post-traumatic stress disorder, coronary atherosclerosis, and mortality. *Am J Cardiol.* 2011;108(1):29-33.

30.   Gros DF, Frueh BC, Magruder KM. Prevalence and features of panic disorder and comparison to posttraumatic stress disorder in VA primary care. *Gen Hosp Psychiatry.* 2011;33(5):482-8.

31.   Yaffe K, Vittinghoff E, Lindquist K, et al. Posttraumatic stress disorder and risk of dementia among US veterans. *Arch Gen Psychiatry.* 2010;67(6):608-13.

32.   Pietrzak RH, Goldstein RB, Southwick SM, Grant BF. Physical health conditions associated with posttraumatic stress disorder in U.S. older adults: results from wave 2 of the National Epidemiologic Survey on Alcohol and Related Conditions. *J Am Geriatr Soc.* 2012;60(2):296-303.

33.   Calhoun PS, McDonald SD, Guerra VS, et al. Clinical utility of the Primary Care-PTSD Screen among U.S. veterans who served since September 11, 2001. *Psychiatry Res.* 2010 30;178(2):330-5.

34.   Cohen BE, Gima K, Bertenthal D, Kim S, Marmar CR, Seal KH. Mental health diagnoses and utilization of VA non-mental health medical services among returning Iraq and Afghanistan veterans. *J Gen Intern Med.* 2010;25(1):18-24.

35.   Zen AL, Whooley MA, Zhao S, Cohen BE. Post-traumatic stress disorder is associated with poor health behaviors: findings from the heart and soul study. *Health Psychol.* 2012;31(2):194-201.

36.   Management of Post-Traumatic Stress Working Group. *VA/DoD clinical practice guideline for management of post-traumatic stress, version 2.0.* Department of Veterans Affairs and Department of Defense; 2010. Available at: www.healthquality.va.gov/ptsd/cpg_PTSD-FULL-201011612.pdf. Accessed January 18, 2013.

37.   Spoont MR, Murdoch M, Hodges J, Nugent S. Treatment receipt by veterans after a PTSD diagnosis in PTSD, mental health, or general medical clinics. *Psychiatr Serv.* 2010;61(1):58-63.

38.   Wang PS, Berglund P, Olfson M, Pincus HA, Wells KB, Kessler RC. Failure and delay in initial treatment contact after first onset of mental disorders in the National Comorbidity Survey Replication. *Arch Gen Psychiatry.* 2005;62(6):603-13.

39.   Blake DD, Weathers FW, Nagy LM, et al. The development of a Clinician-Administered PTSD Scale. *J Trauma Stress.* 1995;8(1):75-90.

40.   First MB, Spitzer RL, Gibbon M, Williams JBW. *Structured Clinical Interview for DSM-IV Axis Disorders.* Washington, DC: American Psychiatric Association; 1997.

41.   Sheehan DV, Lecrubier Y, Sheehan KH, et al. The Mini-International Neuropsychiatric Interview (M.I.N.I.): the development and validation of a structured diagnostic psychiatric interview for DSM-IV and ICD-10. *J Clin Psychiatry.* 1998;59 Suppl 20:22-33.

42.   Foa E, Riggs D, Dancu C, Rothbaum B. Reliability and validity of a brief instrument for assessing post-traumatic stress disorder. *J Trauma Stress.* 1993;6:459-74.

43.   Breslau N, Peterson EL, Kessler RC, Schultz LR. Short screening scale for DSM-IV posttraumatic stress disorder. *Am J Psychiatry.* 1999;156(6):908-11.

44.   Meltzer-Brody S, Churchill E, Davidson JR. Derivation of the SPAN, a brief diagnostic screening test for post-traumatic stress disorder. *Psychiatry Res.* 1999;88(1):63-70.

45.   Davidson JR, Book SW, Colket JT, et al. Assessment of a new self-rating scale for post-traumatic stress disorder. *Psychol Med.* 1997;27(1):153-60.

46.   Weathers F, Litz B, Herman D, Huska J, Keane T. *The PTSD Checklist (PCL): Reliability, validity, and diagnostic utility.* San Antonio , TX: Annual Convention of the International Society for Traumatic Stress Studies; 1993.

47.   Andrykowski MA, Cordova MJ, Studts JL, Miller TW. Posttraumatic stress disorder after treatment for breast cancer: prevalence of diagnosis and use of the PTSD Checklist-Civilian Version (PCL-C) as a screening instrument. *J Consult Clin Psychol.* 1998;66(3):586-90.

48.   Bliese PD, Wright KM, Adler AB, Cabrera O, Castro CA, Hoge CW. Validating the primary care posttraumatic stress disorder screen and the posttraumatic stress disorder checklist with soldiers returning from combat. *J Consult Clin Psychol.* 2008;76(2):272-81.

49.   Lang AJ, Stein MB. An abbreviated PTSD checklist for use as a screening instrument in primary care. *Behav Res Ther.* 2005;43(5):585-94.

50.   Houston JP, Kroenke K, Davidson JR, et al. PDI-4A: an augmented provisional screening instrument assessing 5 additional common anxiety-related diagnoses in adult primary care patients. *Postgrad Med.* 2011;123(5):89-95.

51.   Means-Christensen AJ, Sherbourne CD, Roy-Byrne PP, Craske MG, Stein MB. Using five questions to screen for five common mental disorders in primary care: diagnostic accuracy of the Anxiety and Depression Detector. *Gen Hosp Psychiatry.* 2006;28(2):108-18.

52.   Spitzer RL, Kroenke K, Williams JB, Lowe B. A brief measure for assessing generalized
       anxiety disorder: the GAD-7. *Arch Int Med.* 2006;166(10):1092-7.

53.   Dobie DJ, Kivlahan DR, Maynard C, et al. Screening for post-traumatic stress disorder in
       female Veteran's Affairs patients: validation of the PTSD checklist. *Gen Hosp Psychiatry.*
       2002;24(6):367-74.

54.   Lang AJ, Laffaye C, Satz LE, Dresselhaus TR, Stein MB. Sensitivity and specificity of
       the PTSD checklist in detecting PTSD in female veterans in primary care. *J Trauma
       Stress.* 2003;16(3):257-64.

55.   Meltzer-Brody S, Hartmann K, Miller WC, Scott J, Garrett J, Davidson J. A brief
       screening instrument to detect posttraumatic stress disorder in outpatient gynecology.
       Obstet Gynecol. 2004;104(4):770-6.

56.   Walker EA, Newman E, Dobie DJ, Ciechanowski P, Katon W. Validation of the PTSD
       checklist in an HMO sample of women. *Gen Hosp Psychiatry.* 2002;24(6):375-80.

APPENDIX A. SEARCH STRATEGIES

I. Ovid MEDLINE

Search Strategy:

1   exp mass screening/ or screen*.mp.

2   exp Stress Disorders, Post-Traumatic/

3   (posttraumatic stress or posttraumatic stress disorder* or post-traumatic stress disorder* or ptsd).mp.

4   combat disorder*.mp. or exp Combat Disorders/)

5   or/2-4

6   1 and 5

7   limit 6 to (english language and humans and yr="1981 -Current")

II. PILOTS Database

Search textword "screen*"

With Limits:
English language
1980 -2012

And Descriptor categories:
"self report instruments, adults" or "self report instruments", "ptsd assessment instruments", "dissociation assessment instruments", "acute stress disorder assessment instruments", "assessment instruments" or "assessment"

APPENDIX B. STUDY SELECTION AND DATA EXTRACTION FORM

Title of Study					Check if Background paper ☐

Journal			First Author	Year 2004	Inclusion Eligibility? Y N

Screening Tool	PCL (version)	PDS	Penn Inv	IES	DTI	DES	Miss. Scale	SPAN	IDCL	PC-PTSD	Other

Base Rate of PTSD:

Response Rates: Screening Sample: _____ Interview Sample: _____

Scoring Stats	Cut-Point(s)	Sensitivity (%)	Specificity (%)	PPV	NPV	+LR	-LR	ROCd'	ROC c-stat (AUC)	Other Outcomes

Diagnostic Measure		Administration
Clinician-Administered PTSD Scale (CAPS)		Face-to-Face
MINI International Neuropsychiatric Interview		
Comprehensive international diagnostic interview (CIDI)		Telephone
Diagnostic Interview Schedule (DIS)		
The Structured Clinical Interview for DSM-IV Disorders (SCID-I).		Telehealth

Notes: (e.g., study design different from single cohort, Info on ease of administration, unique scoring method, etc.)

Special Samples	Women trauma Veterans Medical Substance Abuse Age 60+ Vietnam only TBI Minorities OEF/OIF Sexual Other (note)

QUADAS Eval

Sample broadly representative of those who would be screened? Y N

Time b/w screen and dx interview: _____ months
Is it considered "concurrent"? Y N

Did whole/ random sample have dx interview?
Whole   Random   (%?)
Random Group Different from Total Group? Y N
Were diagnostic interviews conducted blindly? Y N
Was screen cut score confirmed on a separate or split sample? Y N
Was relevant clinical data available for interpretation of screen (like would be in clinic)? Y N
Were *reasons for* withdrawals or refusals in the study explained? Y N

+LR= sensitivity/(1-specificity)   **-LR**= (1-sensitivity)/specificity
Good test= LR+ of at least 2.0 and LR- of 0.5 or less.

	Diagnostic (Gold Standard) Test	
	Positive	Negative
Screening Test — Positive:	a (true positive)	b (false positive)	PPV=a/(a+b)
Screening Test — Negative:	c (false negative)	d (true negative)	NPV=d/(c+d)
	Sens=a/(a+c)	Spec=d/(b+d)

Psychometric Notes

APPENDIX C. LEVELS OF EVIDENCE

Based on Criteria for the Rational Clinical Examination Series (Simel 2008)[7]

Level I Evidence

Independent, blind comparison of sign or symptom results with a "gold standard" of anatomy, physiology, diagnosis, or prognosis among a large number of consecutive patients suspected of having the target condition.

Independent: neither the test result nor the gold standard result are used to select patients for the study.

Blind: test and gold standard each applied and interpreted without knowledge of the result of the other.

Gold Standard: the results of biopsy, angiography, autopsy, xray, sonogram, physiologic study, follow-up, therapeutic response, etc. that establish the true anatomy, physiology, diagnosis or outcome of the target condition.

Target Condition: the anatomic or physiologic state, disease, syndrome, prognosis or therapeutic response that the sign or symptom is designed to identify.

Large Numbers: sufficient numbers of patients to have narrow confidence limits on the resulting sensitivity, specificity, or likelihood ratio.

Level II Evidence

Independent, blind comparison of sign or symptom results with a "gold standard" among a small number of consecutive patients suspected of having the target condition.

Small Number: insufficient numbers of patients to have narrow confidence limits on the resulting sensitivity, specificity, or likelihood ratio. (N.B. You should note that the definition of "small" is relative and depends on the size of all extant studies. For example, if you have several studies of many hundreds of patients, then a study of only 80 patients might be considered small.)

Level III Evidence

Independent, blind comparison of signs and symptoms with a "gold standard" among non-consecutive patients suspected of having the target condition. The short-coming here is restricting the study sample to a subset of patients who both underwent and generated definitive results on both the sign or symptom and the application of the gold standard. The results over-estimate accuracy.

Level IV Evidence

Non-independent comparison of signs and symptoms with a "gold standard" among "grab" samples of patients who obviously have the target condition plus, perhaps, normal individuals. In addition to the selection bias of Level III, these studies restrict their samples to the obvious, "black or white" presentations (sometimes even selected on the basis of their gold standard result) that don't need a clinical examination (other than pattern recognition), and exclude the "shades of gray" that comprise the clinical spectrum of early as well as late, mild as well as severe, and other but commonly confused conditions. The results greatly over-estimate accuracy.

Level V Evidence

Non-independent comparisons of signs and symptoms with a standard of uncertain validity (which may even "incorporate" the sign or symptom result in its definition) among "grab" samples of patients plus, perhaps, normals. In addition to the biases of Level IV, these studies often include the sign or symptom result as part of a "lead standard," resulting in a self-fulfilling prophesy. The results extravagantly over-estimate accuracy.

APPENDIX D. PEER REVIEW COMMENTS/AUTHOR RESPONSES

REVIEWER COMMENT	RESPONSE
1. Are the objectives, scope, and methods for this review clearly described?	
Yes.	
1. This is an excellent and comprehensive review with a wealth of very useful information.	1. Thank you
2. The objective of the report appears to be a literature synthesis of the feasibility and diagnostic accuracy of PTSD screening tools for primary care settings. This could be slightly clarified in the introduction, rather than the broad statement on literature on screening tools in general, since issues of screening effectiveness and clinical efficiency appear to be beyond the scope of the report.	2. We have modified the statement of the objective of the review.
3. For the most part, the key questions are clearly stated, but could avoid using "etc." in KQ #1 and 2, and instead clearly state the specific characteristics reviewed, and for KQ#2, list the specific psychometric properties of interest. I am not sure that the implementability issue fits better in KQ#2 than it would in KQ#1 or as a separate question, since that information is reviewed separately on page 18, and does not map to the levels of evidence framework used to evaluate the question of diagnostic accuracy (psychometric properties and utility) in KQ#2.	3. We have modified KQ1 and 2 as suggested. We agree that the implementation processes of screening would have best been covered in a separate question and have done so to improve clarity of the findings.
4. Explanation and application of levels of evidence need to be clearer, especially in the discrimination of levels II and III:	4. The descriptions of levels of evidence were taken from instructions for preparing a Rational Clinical Examination article.
a. The description of the shortcoming for level III, "patients who both underwent and generated definitive results on both the sign and symptom and the application of the gold standard" is not clear. I am wondering if this is an allusion to the verification bias where follow-up or administration of one part of the testing protocol is dependent of results from a prior part of the testing protocol (e.g. administering the gold standard first, and then the screen to all cases but only a sample of controls, as described in Simel). I'm also wondering if this may be an editing glitch, since this text is repeated in the summary for level IV, and this kind of non-independence would be more of a Level IV issue.	4a. We agree that the shortcoming for Level III is verification bias – selection of patients for verification rather than inclusion of consecutive patients. We also agree that the section of text was mistakenly repeated in the summary
b. The key element that can take a study from Level II to Level III is the use of non-consecutive patients that are selected on the basis of some factor other than eligibility for screening that would result in a non-representative sample and introduce bias. Such results do not reliably over estimate accuracy, as stated on p. 48. The effect of the bias will be due to how the sample was selected and the ways in which they differ from the target population. Examples cited in the STARD guidelines include: exclusion of patients with comorbid conditions or symptoms that could adversely affect test accuracy but would likely be present in the target population; studies in specialty settings where the spectrum of symptom expression is narrowed; or just non-consecutive and non-random selection of the sample. I would then assume that pronounced violations of sampling assumptions, such as case control studies, would be graded at Level IV.	4b. We agree that selection bias is one of the main differences between Level II and Level III studies. We have clarified our application of these ratings in Appendix F.
5. The discussion of each screen under KQ#2 could be more complete and detailed. Not all psychometric properties included in the articles are consistently reported, including key indicators of diagnostic accuracy such as likelihood ratios and (if provided) post-test odds of a positive test. If only sensitivity and specificity are reported, it is important to include the prevalence of PTSD in the sample. This may be a minor issue, since most (but not all) of this information is in Table 5, but it is not clear why some specific statistics are pulled out in the text and that the type of statistics discussed are not completely consistent across measures, so the reader does not get a clear critique of the state of the evidence for each screener.	5. We have now made the text more consistent throughout.
Yes	Thank you

REVIEWER COMMENT	RESPONSE
Yes and No Yes, the objectives of the review are clearly described through the three key questions: Question 1: What tools are used to screen for PTSD in primary care settings, and what are their characteristics (length, format, etc)? Question 2: What are the psychometric properties and utility of the screening (operating characteristics) and their implementability (ease of administration) in primary care clinics? Question 3: Do the psychometric properties and utility of each of the screening tools differ according to age, gender, race/ethnicity, substance abuse or other comorbidities? Yes, the scope of the review is on screening tools used and validated in primary care. No, the methods for the review are not always logical, accurate or clearly described 1. Study selection a. Rationale for why studies outside of the US were excluded was not provided. Discussion of how Veterans in VA primary care may differ from civilians in primary care was not addressed. Perhaps there are reasons why screening practices/recommendations might differ in VA versus civilian primary care. Greater rationale for the inclusion/ exclusion of studies seems warranted.	1. We have addressed these points in the report. 1a. We included only studies done in the United States because of greater relevance to the care of US Veterans. There were no studies that compared screen efficiency or effectiveness across both Veteran and non-Veteran samples. It may be that a given screen performs better in one population vs. another or for PTSD associated with one type of trauma vs. another; however, given the absence of evidence this would be purely speculative on our part. Available evidence suggests that PTSD is under-recognized in non-Veteran primary care settings (c.f. Graves, 2011) suggesting that, from a healthcare system perspective, screening for PTSD might also facilitate further mental health evaluation and treatment among non-Veterans assuming available mental health resources. As to whether screening practices/recommendations do or should differ in Veteran vs. non-Veteran primary care settings is a matter of policy and resource availability not screen characteristics and so is beyond the scope of this review. We have clarified the rationale for inclusion/exclusion of studies.
b. Why were screens included that did not include PTSD items (e.g., GAD-7)? Was study selection based on administration of a PTSD gold standard in a primary care setting? If yes, other non-PTSD screens may need to be considered in the review (e.g., GHQ)	1b. We state that we included screens for multiple psychiatric disorders or multiple anxiety disorders if there was a study that investigated the ability of the screen to identify PTSD in a primary care setting. No other screens identified in our literature search process were eligible for inclusion.
c. If studies with fewer than 50 participants were excluded, why was the Lange et al, (2003) study included? There were only 49 women interviewed with the gold standard interview.	1c. We excluded studies with fewer than 50 patients in the screening population.
d. There appears to be an assumption that gold standards are equivalent. This may not be an accurate assumption. Furthermore, it seems important to recognize that there are different scoring algorithms within gold standards. For example, there are at least 9 different scoring rules for the CAPS and the selection of one over another will surely impact diagnostic accuracy. Granted, scoring rules are rarely presented in studies, but the importance of this should not be overlooked.	1d. We identified the gold standard diagnostic tool used in each study and noted where scoring for the gold standard differed from the scoring method described in Table 1. We agree that different gold standard instruments or scoring rules could alter the findings in a given study. As the reviewer notes, scoring rules are rarely presented in studies, as was true in the vast majority of studies included in this review. While we do not think that variation in gold standard instrumentation or scoring would appreciably alter the overall findings of the review, we have included a statement of that possibility in our limitations section.

Screening for Post-Traumatic Stress Disorder (PTSD) in Primary Care: A Systematic Review

REVIEWER COMMENT	RESPONSE
2. Screen/study description a. The PC-PTSD does not include a stem that asks about traumatic events. This is inaccurately reflected in the description of the measure: "Respondents are asked about symptoms experienced in response to a traumatic event in the past month" (p. 13)	2a. This has been clarified.
b. The SPAN was not validated with a primary care sample in the original Meltzer-Brody study. It was "developed in a psychiatry clinic for the purpose of detecting PTSD in psychiatric populations with PTSD prevalence around 50%" (p14). Yes, it was argued that it could be used in settings with a lower prevalence, like primary care, and yes, it was tested in primary care setting in the Yeager et al., study, but it was not developed/validated in primary care.	2b. We include the SPAN because there was a study that tested it in primary care setting as noted above.
c. The review correctly recognizes that there are three different versions of the PCL, and three different scoring options (p.14). All three versions of the PCL are represented in the studies reviewed, and information on scoring algorithms is often missing. The review treats the PCL as a single screen and does not mention how scoring options may impact diagnostic accuracy. This seems problematic for the accuracy and validity of the review.	2c. We have clarified which version of the PCL was used in each study. However, while there are different versions of the PCL and different scoring approaches to the instrument (e.g., symptoms/symptom cluster, total score, etc.), we believe that the importance of these differences is greatly attenuated when the PCL is used as a screening tool rather than as a diagnostic tool, a tool to assess symptom change in treatment, or as a means to estimate population prevalence rates (see Wilkins et al., 2011). Because the function of a screening tool is to identify individuals in need of further evaluation, all PTSD screening tools have lower discriminability than one would expect from a diagnostic tool. The more relevant scoring issue is cut-score, and we made efforts to include information about multiple cut-scores when studies provided that information. Accordingly, we do not feel that the accuracy or the validity of the review has been compromised.
d. As previously mentioned, it is unclear why the GAD-7/GAD-2 is included in the review. The screen does not include any PTSD items.	2d. As stated above, we included screens if there was a study that investigated the ability of the screen to identify PTSD in a primary care setting. Although the GAD-7 or GAD-2 may not be specific to PTSD, whether it performs better or worse than a PTSD-specific screen was an empirical question we thought worth considering given an appropriate gold standard and study design.
3. Table 3: summary of screens used in primary care a. It is not clear which study was used to report on test-retest reliability	3a. References have been added to Table (see footnotes).
b. Although scoring may be the same for briefer versions of the PCL, test-retest reliability cannot be assumed to be the same.	3b. We have noted this on Table 3.
c. Should internal consistency be presented as well?	3c. Internal consistency has been noted on Table 3 where reported (see footnotes).
Yes and No Some things are clearly described, but further justification is needed for the decisions the authors chose to make, e.g., to include studies of non-Veterans given the target audience of this report. The absence of this content makes it difficult to judge the statement on p. 30 that there is no information as to whether a given screen performs better in Veteran or non-Veteran samples.	We have clarified the inclusion and exclusion criteria. Our literature search yielded no studies comparing the performance of screening tests in Veteran and non-Veteran samples. We have now highlighted results of studies in Veterans in the discussion to make it more relevant for the target audience of the report.

REVIEWER COMMENT	RESPONSE
Yes. As stated on page 1, the premise of screening for PTSD is "to facilitate mental health treatment engagement 1) earlier in the course of the illness and 2) to engage patients in treatment who might otherwise not be identified..." For this purpose, the report undertakes to identify PTSD screeners for primary care (pc) settings and evaluate them, using the published literature. Three questions were formulated, which address evidence on the utility (and relative utility) of available scales. The questions and the methodology to answer them are perhaps too narrowly formulated. This is especially the case when one becomes aware of the fact that the studies that have evaluated PTSD screeners in pc have not evaluated the impact of screenings in engaging mental health workers more effectively, in terms of reaching patients who would not be identified. As a result, the report is a technical evaluation of the studies that evaluated PTSD screeners in pc: their design, analysis, etc. The lion share of the work—the evaluation of screening (by any means) for mental health delivery, and the outcome in terms of improving health— remains to be done.	Thank you. We agree, that there is important work that remains to be done involving the impact of screen use on the delivery of mental health care and on health outcomes. We included this in our recommendations.
2. Is there any indication of bias in our synthesis of the evidence?	
No. I do not see any evidence of bias.	Thank you
No	Thank you
Yes and No A. Not sure about bias, but there are some problematic statements about the PC-PTSD and PCL. 1. Appendix E: Evidence Tables (Prins et al., 2003) a. The PC-PTSD was evaluated in one VA Health Care Facility, not two different VA's in California. b. The CAPS was administered in person, not over the phone c. As noted in the Evidence Table, the use of blind interviews was "not reported". The assumption was made, however, that interviewers were not blind (versus not reported), and the study was given a level IV rating. Although not clear from the original study, interviewers were indeed blind. Perhaps "not-reported" findings can be followed-up rather than assumed to be negative.	1a. This has been corrected. 1b. Thank you for clarifying this. 1c. Thank you for providing this additional information. Given this clarification, we have now determined that this study should have a rating of Level III.
2. Freedy et al., 2010 a. Similar to Prins et al., 2003 -- It is assumed that interviewers were not blind to the screen results because they were administered on the same day as the diagnostic interview. But, what was the order of administration? Did interviewers know how to interpret screen results (cutoff scores for screens)?	2a. We assumed that interviews were not blind not because of their timing relative to administration of the screen, but rather because non-blind evaluations may be biased (similar to RCTs), and so the absence of a clear statement indicating that diagnostic interviews were conducted blindly in most cases means that they were not. However, as suggested by this reviewer, we sent an email to Dr. Freedy requesting further information, but have not received a response in the more than one month since the email was sent.
3. PCL a. The PCL version used in the Yeager et all study is not clear. In the study, the PCL is described as "a series of 17 questions about symptoms or signs of PTSD resulting from military experiences taking place within the past month" . This suggests that the PCL-M was used.	3a. We have clarified that no version was specified in this study.
b. The PCL version used in the Prins et al., 2003 study is also not clear. However, a correction to the article was published with clear reference to the PCL-S (Prins & Ouimette, 2004, Primary Care Psychiatry, 9, p151). The review also states that 124 "woman" [sic], were screened and interviewed. That is incorrect, 167 participants completed both the PCL-S and the PC-PTSD.	3b. We have clarified that the PCL-S was used in this study. We have replaced the data from the original paper with the data presented in the Corrigendum.
No. The report gives no indication of bias in any of the decision or text.	Thank you.
No	Thank you.

Screening for Post-Traumatic Stress Disorder (PTSD) in Primary Care: A Systematic Review

REVIEWER COMMENT	RESPONSE
3. Are there any published or unpublished studies that we may have overlooked?	
Yes. There is some evidence that the PC-PTSD performs adequately in VA substance use populations (p. 37, item 3). See Kimerling et al., (2006) Addictive Behaviors 31(11).	We are familiar with the Kimerling (2006) study but did not include it in this review because the study sample was that of patients who were receiving substance abuse treatment and not those presenting in primary care clinics.
No. Question whether it was necessary to include studies done on MH population and instruments that are not specific screens for PTSD – specifically the GAD-7	As noted previously, we included screens if there was a study that investigated the ability of the screen to identify PTSD in a primary care setting.
Yes For excellent reviews of the PCL, including the importance of spectrum effects (e.g., age, race, etc) bias, and prevalence, please see: 1. McDonald, S.D. & Calhoun, P.S. (2010). The diagnostic accuracy of the PTSD Checklist: A critical review. Clinical Psychology Review. doi:10:1016/j.cpr.2010.06.012. 2. Wilkins, K.C., Lang, A.J., & Norman, S.B. (2011). Synthesis of the psychometric properties of the PTSD Checklist (PCL) military, civilian, and specific versions. Depression and Anxiety. doi: 10.1002/da.20837.	Thank you for sharing these references. These reviews provide excellent background information on the PCL but do not focus on studies conducted in primary care.
Yes The report is so comprehensive that I think it will surprise readers in its presentation of studies they may not know of. However, it could be even more complete in several respects: 1. There is a corrigendum to the Prins et al. 2003 study that reports critically important information about the PCL. There were significant errors in the 2003 report due to a software problem regarding the handling of missing data. The data reported on the PCL need to be based on the 2004 correction. 2. A paper by Calhoun and colleagues (2010) comparing the SPAN and the PC-PTSD may have been overlooked.	Thank you. We have addressed your concerns. 1. We have updated the report based on the Corrigendum. 2. We reviewed this excellent paper but it did not meet our inclusion criteria. Subjects in that study were part of the Mid-Atlantic MIRECC post-deployment registry and consisted of Veterans who served in the military after to September 11, 2001. According to the authors, "Eligible Veterans were recruited through mailings, advertisements, and clinician referrals." As such, it was not eligible for this review. 3. We did not include studies because of missing information. As noted in the Literature Flow (Figure 1) studies were excluded if the study setting, population, or purpose did not meet our inclusion criteria.
3. In meta-analysis it is common to ask authors for data needed to include the paper in the analysis. Was there any attempt to contact investigators for information that could have allowed an excluded paper to be included? If not, I recommend that the authors use this strategy if it possibly could yield additional studies to include in the review	
No. No overlooked study on screening scales in primary care.	Thank you.
4. Please write any additional suggestions or comments below. If applicable, please indicate the page and line numbers from the draft report.	
Future directions #6 is an important point, and the authors may want to specifically refer to the need for studies of screening effectiveness in VA.	Thank you for this suggestion. We have now made our recommendations more specific.
P. 1: first paragraph: I don't think the screening is meant to "Identify PTSD," or to facilitate treatment engagement so much as to identify Veterans who need further evaluation and possibly treatment for PTSD. Similar issue in the more detailed paragraph near end of page 5. Screening is not necessarily correlated with reducing delays for treatment – in fact, in VA the typical concern from PTSD teams is that PC refers too many patients because of a positive screen, thus tying up the resources needed to reduce access delays (though screening can lead to earlier diagnosis and an opportunity for intervention earlier in the course of an individual's illness). These issues do receive some discussion in the "clinical consideration" paragraph on page 38.	Thank you for this feedback. We clarified the statement on page to indicate that screens are intended to facilitate detection of a condition (in this case PTSD), not to identify it directly. We agree that screening is not correlated with treatment; however, the purpose of screening programs is to increase the rate of treatment, particularly among those early in the course of the illness as you note. The concern you raise about too many patients having positive screens and the effect of this on limited clinical resources is an important one. This suggests that from a clinical standpoint the screen used by VA is too sensitive as it is currently employed; however, altering the screen cut score to address this has clear policy implications that may be difficult to resolve.

REVIEWER COMMENT	RESPONSE
1. "Screening tools that focus on evaluating traumatic experiences are not likely to be clinically useful given the high population prevalence of traumatic events and the much lower conditional probability of developing PTSD (IOM, Breslau, Wang)" p.36 a. True, but the diagnostic precision of screens that include a trauma exposure item versus those that don't has not been empirically established. Perhaps inclusion of a trauma exposure question will decrease the number of false positives in primary care. Future research could compare screens with and without a trauma probe. b. Does this statement suggest that screening for military sexual trauma is not warranted?	1a. The statement that you reference was meant to clarify the scope of the review. On the other hand, we agree that whether screen performance would be improved with inclusion of a traumatic exposure item(s) is a worthy empirical question.
2. "Very short screens (i.e., one or two items) performed less well than longer screens with positive likelihood ratios less than 3.0, making them less clinically useful" p. 3 PLUS, "Screens not specific to PTSD but for which there was a study that evaluated the ability of the screen to detect PTSD performed less well than those that focused on the detection of PTSD exclusively" p.37 a. Combined, these argue against the use of the SIPS or multi-purpose screens with only 1 or 2 items relevant to PTSD. b. So, moderate to longer PTSD screens seem to be better but the threshold for acceptable length is not clear. If "successful screening programs utilize instruments that are simple, valid, precise, and acceptable both clinically and socially" (p. 1), the remaining PTSD screens should be evaluated along these dimensions. For example, future research needs to determine preference and ease of administration based on number of items, reading level, response format, etc	1b. No. It simply clarifies the scope of the review. 2a. We agree with the reviewer's conclusion that the available evidence suggests that screens longer than 2 items perform better. 2b. We did not find any information that any of the screening tools used in the studies cited in this review were unacceptable to patients or administrators. The longest screening tool (27 items) was reported to take patients only 10 minutes to complete, suggesting that none of the screens would be administratively burdensome. However, given the absence of comparative information about patient or provider preferences regarding screening tools, further research would be needed to make definitive statements about these issues.
3. "However, there were no high quality studies examining the performance of the PC-PTSD in a primary care setting" p.37 a. Perhaps Freedy, Prins, and Gore can be contacted for clarification on the QUADAS ratings, and subsequent changes made to level of evidence.	3a. We have updated the information from one of the studies mentioned and adjusted the quality assessment. We contacted the author of another study for clarification but did not receive a response. We did not find anything requiring clarification in the third study.
The report has the potential to be an important guide for both practice and research. It is well done is so many respects but it could be enhanced by additions to the text and tables. It also needs to be cleaned for typos, some of which are important (e.g., on p. 20 the paragraph on the PCL says in one place that there were 2 studies and in another that there were 3, Table 4 shows 3, and the paragraph mentions an additional study by Kimerling (2006) that does not appear in the table). Specific recommendations are as follows: 1. More detail is needed about how the quality assessment ratings were determined. Although detail is provide in the Appendices, I could not make the crosswalk between the QUADAS evaluation questions in Appendix B, Appendix C, the 5 criteria listed for each study in Appendix E, and the level of evidence rating. In fact, I don't see the clear connection between the QUADAS criteria and the QUADAS questions in Appendix B. For example, in QUADAS, representativeness is about whether the full range of patients to whom a test would be applied was included in the sample. It appears that sample representativeness—and not spectrum inclusiveness—was more important in evaluating studies for the report. The fact that a study had one site is mentioned in a couple places, even though this is not relevant to evaluating quality according to the QUADAS or RSES systems. RCES level 1 evidence requires that neither the test result nor gold standard was used to select patients. Yeager's study, which was rated at the highest level, is mentioned as being a random sample of participants from 4 sites, whereas Andrykowski's study is described as "women in remission from breast cancer." Note that there is a typo in Appendix C and elsewhere in the text: it should be "Rational" not "Rationale" Clinical Examination Series.	Thank you. We have corrected the typos and clarified the additional studies cited in the paragraph on the PC-PTSD. 1. Thank you for pointing this out. We have now included an additional table in our appendices (Appendix F) that clarifies the relationship between the individual QUADAS ratings and the overall Level of Evidence ratings. Now that we have included the crosswalk table in the report, we hope that study ratings have been clarified. The Andrykowski study was rated as a Level IV because the diagnostic interviews were not conducted blind to patient screening status. We have corrected the typo.

REVIEWER COMMENT	RESPONSE
2. Figure 1 was illegible when the document was printed, even though it appeared fine on the screen. Also, I recommend providing the N for each reason the 122 excluded studies ruled out.	2. We have added the number of studies for each exclusion reason.
3. In Table 3 it would help to know the test-retest interval for each study.	3. We have added this information to Table 3 (see footnotes).
4. Table 4 should specify the gold-standard measure used for each study and if relevant how it was scored, e.g., the "1/2" rule for the CAPS.	4. We have added the gold standard measure to Table 4. Studies did not typically report how the measure was scored.
5. For Key Question 2, the amount of detail in the text about studies varies unsystematically. For example, there was no information on p. 20 about the sample used in the Prins 2003 study and a lot of information on p. 22 about the sample used in the Dobie 2002 study.	5. We have reviewed this and standardized the amount of text.
6. On p. 21 only 2 SPAN studies were discussed but the Table 4 lists 3. Freedy 2010 is excluded.	6. We have added Freedy 2010 to the discussion of the SPAN studies.
7. Caution is needed regarding the inferences that are drawn when relevant information is missing. For example, and perhaps most notably, on p. 22, the report says that it is unclear whether CAPS interviewers were blind to PCL scores in the Prins 2003 study but elsewhere the report specifically states that lack of blinding was a major flaw of this study. Lack of information about blinding is not the same thing as lack of blinding. Regardless, things like this are so important that it is worth asking authors for missing information.	7. As noted above, we have obtained information from one author and another author did not respond to our inquiry.

8. Table 5 is difficult to read. The use of shading to indicate different screens does not provide enough clarity or distinctiveness. For example, the authors could use a separate leftmost column to indicate the screen, with the study information in a column to the right:
 	
Screen   Author/Year   Cutpoints
Breslau   Freedy 2010   xx
    Kimerling 2006   xx
PC-PTSD   Freedy 2010   xx
    Gore 2008   xx
	8. Thank you for the suggestion. We have modified the table.

9. Given that the report includes studies of both Veterans and non-Veterans, can any more be said about whether findings might generalize from one population to the other?	9. A comment about Veterans vs. non-Veterans has been added to the discussion.
10. Given that the PC-PTSD is currently used for screening in both VA and DoD settings, can any more be said other than a recommendation for a study comparing it with other screening instruments?	10. Our primary recommendation is for VA (and DoD) to evaluate whether use of the screen has improved health outcomes for Veterans and to examine the impact of its use on the healthcare system.
11. I recommend rewording recommendation 3 on p. 38. There is plenty of evidence about how screening tools work in the presence of other comorbidities because comorbidity is the rule rather than the exception in PTSD. What is missing is information about whether there is differential performance as a function of comorbidity.	11. Thank you for the suggestion. We have reworded the statement and clarified our point.
12. The relevance of recommendation 4 is unclear or perhaps is not clearly worded. There is evidence about depression and anxiety screening in Veterans.	12. We agree that this point needs rewording as well, and incorporated the intended point elsewhere.
It would be of interest to have a review of the literature on screening among Veterans of other countries. Can we learn anything from this literature? Can we learn anything from DoD screening?	We chose not to include DoD studies because screening among active duty service members is complicated by limited confidentiality, potential deleterious effect of mental health diagnoses on military careers, and greater levels of stigma related to mental health conditions compared to that seen in non-active duty populations.
5. Are there any clinical performance measures, programs, quality improvement measures, patient care services, or conferences that will be directly affected by this report? If so, please provide detail.	
Not at this time. PC-PTSD followed by PCL when indicated is current measure and this report is unlikely to affect that.	Thank you
1. It seems like data from the PCMHI office may be able to address the impact of PTSD screening on referrals to co-located care or specialty care (i.e., access to care measure). And, with the new OEF4 performance measure, it might be possible to look at screening and engagement with treatment (8 sessions within 14 weeks).	1. We agree that evaluating the impact of screening implementation on service utilization is an important area that should be explored.
2. DSM5 is around the corner. The content validity and predictive validity of PTSD screens will need to be evaluated against these new diagnostic criteria.	2. We agree and have now commented on the upcoming DSM-5 modifications.

REVIEWER COMMENT	RESPONSE
The performance measure for PTSD screening is simply an indicator of whether screening has occurred, so I think this answer is no.	Thank you
6. Please provide any recommendations on how this report can be revised to more directly address or assist implementation needs.	
1. Perhaps more focused statements can be made about how the review can inform policy, guide services, support performance measures, and direct future research. For example: a. Although additional research is needed on what screen is best for detecting PTSD in VA primary care, there are good reasons to screen for PTSD in VA (see guidelines propose by US Preventive Services Task Force). b. Currently, if a patient screens positive for PTSD, CPRS presents certain follow-up options/services. Indeed, the clinical reminder is not "resolved" until an option is selected. The report would be strengthened by addressing these options and perhaps making recommendations for additional ones.	1a. To our knowledge the USPSTF does not currently recommend routine PTSD screening. However, VA has significant clinical and political impetus for conducting routine PTSD screens on Veterans who use VA services. 1b. Although the requirement to institute a particular clinical reminder may be a result of national VA policy, how the clinical reminders are implemented varies across VISNs. Consequently, it would be less helpful to make specific recommendations about how the performance measure should be resolved. 1c. We agree.
c. As previously noted, the relationship between PTSD screening and access to care, and type of care would enhance implementation needs. 2. For future research, more specific examples of what should be done is needed. For example, a. Which screens (moderate and longer screens?) should be compared in VA primary care clinics and on what dimensions (ease of administration, diagnostic accuracy)? b. How should the impact of spectrum effects be analyzed? Comparing AUC's may not be the best approach.	2a. We do not recommend any particular screening tool since all have their limitations. Specific recommendations for future research are delineated. b. If what the reviewer means by "spectrum effects" is subsyndromal PTSD, then we agree that this would have implications for the criterion of a study. Comparisons of screen AUC's across studies requires a comparable outcome criterion.
With the formal adoption of DSM-5 in May 2013, the relevance of the data based on DSM-IV are unclear. Data obtained from DSM-IV versions may not generalize to DSM-5 versions if and when such data would be available. The authors need to address this issue more directly and incorporate it into their recommendations.	Agreed. We have now included comments about the relevance of the review with respect to DSM-5.

APPENDIX E. EVIDENCE TABLE

Author, Year / Screen	Gold Standard	Screen Sample I. Age, gender, special population II. Response Rate	Interview Sample I. Age, gender, special population II. Response rate	QUADAS Item Ratings I. Representativeness II. Quality of Gold Standard III. Concurrent IV. % Interviewed V. Blind Interviews RCE Level of Evidence
Freedy 2010[11] **Breslau**	CAPS	I. Not reported; required to be ≥18 years old, English speaking, no gross cognitive impairment, medically stable II. 774 of 3728 approached in clinic consented (20.8%); 519 of 774 consented were contacted (67%); telephone interviews done in 411 (11% of those approached in clinic, 53% of those consented, 79% of those contacted for interview)	I. 53% 18-44 years old, 19% 45-54 years old, 19% 55-65 years old, 7% 66-75 years old, 1.2% ≥76 years 83% women 65% white, 32% African American, 3% other 45% married 24% high school education or less II. 100% of those screened	I. No (significant differences in gender and race from clinic population during recruitment period) II. Fair (telephone, experienced survey interviewers) III. Yes IV. 79% of those who were contacted for interview V. No **Level of Evidence: IV**
Kimerling 2006[13] **Breslau**	CAPS	I. Veterans; other screen sample characteristics NR II. 237 of 258 approached (92%) were eligible and completed Breslau scale	I. Veterans Mean age = 52 years (range 22 to 85) 61% women 68% white, 18% African American, 5% Hispanic, 5% Asian/Pacific Islander, 1% Native American, 3% other 44% married 59% employed II. 57% returned for interview (significantly higher percentage of women in participants vs. non-participants)	I. Yes II. Good (in person, trained psychologists) III. Yes, approximately 1 month IV. 57% of those who consented, completed Breslau scale and were eligible V. Yes **Level of Evidence: III**
Freedy 2010[11] **PC-PTSD**	See above			
Gore 2008[10] **PC-PTSD**	PSS-I	I. 21% <30 years; 24% 31-34 years old; 31% 41-50 years old; 16% 51-60 years old; 8% ≥61 years 60% male Recruited from 3 military health system primary care clinics in Washington, DC area (service members, retirees, and family members) II. estimated 87.4% (3234 of approximately 3700 approached) NOTE: participants first administered SIPS; subgroup participated in 2nd phase of study (PC-PTSD and structured clinical interview); unclear if all invited to participate in 2nd phase	I. 24% <30 years, 23% 31-34 years old, 31% 41-50 years old, 18% 51-60 years old, 4% ≥61 years 61% male II. 93% of those who consented to interview (213/229); 6.6% of those screened (213/3234)	I. Unclear; oversampled patients who responded "bothered a little" and "bothered a lot" to single screening question II. Fair (unclear if in-person or telephone, trained mental health professionals) III. Yes IV. 6.6% of those screened V. Yes **Level of Evidence: III**

Author, Year Screen	Gold Standard	Screen Sample I. Age, gender, special population II. Response Rate	Interview Sample I. Age, gender, special population II. Response rate	QUADAS Item Ratings I. Representativeness II. Quality of Gold Standard III. Concurrent IV. % Interviewed V. Blind Interviews RCE Level of Evidence
Prins 2003[9] PC-PTSD	CAPS	I. Not reported; recruited from general medical and women's health clinics at a VA facility in California; required to have no gross cognitive impairment and English speaking II. Number approached for screening not reported	I. Mean age = 52 years* 34.0% male 33% married 43% unemployed 27% high school education or less II. 50% of those who completed screening (167/335); participants repeated the PC-PTSD at the interview NOTE: all screened individuals invited to participate in interview	I. VA sample from 1 VA in California with 50% response rate II. Good (in-person, trained psychologists) III. Yes IV. 50% V. Yes **Level of Evidence: III**
Gore 2008[10] SIPS	See above			
Freedy 2010[11] SPAN	See above			
Meltzer-Brody 2004[55] SPAN	MINI	I. Mean age = 34 years 100% female 43% white, 49% African-American 30% (n=88/292) reported a traumatic event and completed the SPAN II. 76% (292/384 approached)	I. Mean age = 35 years 52% white, 41% African American II. 11% of total sample (32/292) of total sample; 36% of those with trauma who were invited for interview (32/88)	I. Women presenting for annual exam at ob/gyn clinic; n=32 completed interview II. Good (in-person, psychiatrist) III. Not reported IV. 11% of total sample V. Yes **Level of Evidence: III**
Yeager 2007[8] SPAN	CAPS	I. Group 1 - Veterans (male & female) II. 74.1% (888/1198) I. Group 2 - Female Veterans (oversample) II. 69.2% (191/276)	I. 79% male 63% white II. Group 1 - 82% of those who completed screen (728/888) or 61% of those approached (728/1198) Group 2 – 68% of those who completed screen (130/191) or 47% of those approached (130/276) NOTE: completers more likely to be older and Caucasian; final analysis (combining Groups 1 and 2) included only Caucasians and African-Americans (840/1079 or 78% of those who completed screen; 840/1474 or 57% of those approached)	I. Random sample from 4 medical centers in southeastern US II. Good (telephone, trained clinicians) III. Yes, within 2 months IV. 57% of total sample V. Yes **Level of Evidence: I**

Author, Year Screen	Gold Standard	Screen Sample I. Age, gender, special population II. Response Rate	Interview Sample I. Age, gender, special population II. Response rate	QUADAS Item Ratings I. Representativeness II. Quality of Gold Standard III. Concurrent IV. % Interviewed V. Blind Interviews RCE Level of Evidence
Andrykowski 1998[47] PCL	SCID NP PTSD module	I. Mean age = 57 years 95% Caucasian, 4% African-American, 1% Asian-American 22% high school education or less NOTE: all had diagnosis of Stage 0 to IIIA breast cancer, without surgery, chemotherapy, or radiotherapy for 6-72 months, in remission II. 84/107 (79%) consented; 2 later deemed ineligible	I. Same as screen sample II. Same as screen sample NOTE: participants completed PCL-C and SCID NP PTSD during one telephone interview	I. Women in remission from breast cancer II. Fair (telephone, doctoral-level students) III. Yes IV. 100% of those consenting; 77% of those invited V. No **Level of Evidence: IV**
Dobie 2002[53] PCL	CAPS	I. Mean age = 48 years 100% female 75% white, 9% black, 15% other 40% married 35% high school education or less II. 16% of those randomly selected for telephone interview (282/1763); 11% of total pool (282/2545)	I. Same as screening II. Same as screening NOTE: participants were older and more often divorced than eligible non-participants	I. Female Veterans (1 site) II. Good (in-person, clinician) III. Yes IV. 11% of total sample V. Yes **Level of Evidence: III**
Freedy 2010[11] PCL	See above			
Lang 2005[49] PCL	CIDI 2.1	I. Primary care from VA or university-affiliated clinic II. Approximately 60% of patients approached in clinic consented; 275/401 completed PCL-C (69% [65% reported in text]) (returned by mail) NOTE: reported that a randomly selected half of those who completed consent form and short set of instruments in waiting room were selected for diagnostic interview	I. Mean age = 48 years 48% male 57% Caucasian 53% married 23% high school education or less II. 186/401 completed CIDI (46% [44% reported in text]) 154/401 completed PCL-C and CIDI (38% [36.5% reported in text])	I. Primary care clinics (VA or university-affiliated) II. Fair (telephone, licensed psychologist or research assistant) III. Not reported IV. 38% of enrolled V. Yes **Level of Evidence: II**

Author, Year Screen	Gold Standard	Screen Sample I. Age, gender, special population II. Response Rate	Interview Sample I. Age, gender, special population II. Response rate	QUADAS Item Ratings I. Representativeness II. Quality of Gold Standard III. Concurrent IV. % Interviewed V. Blind Interviews RCE Level of Evidence
Lang 2003[54] **PCL**	CIDI	I. 100% female Veterans (1 site) II. 56% agreed to participate and returned questionnaires (221/394) NOTE: 25 of 419 survey packets were undeliverable	I. Mean age = 53 years 82% Caucasian, 12% African-American; 6% other/ unknown 39% married 80% with 9-15 years of education NOTE: interviewed women were older, more likely Caucasian, more likely divorced, separated, or widowed; less likely to be never married II. 87% of those screened willing to be interviewed (192/221); 46% of those approached (192/419) 26% randomly selected for interview (49/192)	I. Female Veterans (1 site) II. Fair (telephone, CIDI designed for lay interviewers) III. Yes, within 1 month IV. 26% (randomly selected, n=49) V. Yes **Level of Evidence: II**
Prins 2003[9] **PCL-S**	See above			
Walker 2002[56] **PCL (not specified)**	CAPS	I. Mean age = 41 years 100% female 79% Caucasian; 6% African-American; 8% Asian, 2% Hispanic, 1% Native-American 51% married 57% college graduates II. Adjusted return rate of 62% (1225/1912 eligible)	I. Not reported II. Overall 21% (261 of 1225 who returned questionnaire) or 14% (261/1912 eligible) – See NOTE NOTE: 305 returned questionnaires and had history of childhood sexual maltreatment, 152 of 204 reached (74%) agreed to interview (or 50% of those with history of maltreatment who returned questionnaires) From sample of 250 without childhood maltreatment, 116 of 155 reached (75%) agreed to interview (or 46% of sample) 7 had missing PCL data; final sample was n=261	I. Women only; random sample of HMO members II. Unclear (Not reported if face-to-face or telephone; qualifications of administrators not reported) III. Yes, within 2 months IV. 50% of those who reported childhood maltreatment; 46% of sample without maltreatment V. Not reported **Level of Evidence: III**
Yeager 2007[8] **PCL (not specified)**	See above			

Evidence-based Synthesis Program

Screening for Post-Traumatic Stress Disorder (PTSD) in Primary Care: A Systematic Review

Author, Year Screen	Gold Standard	Screen Sample I. Age, gender, special population II. Response Rate	Interview Sample I. Age, gender, special population II. Response rate	QUADAS Item Ratings I. Representativeness II. Quality of Gold Standard III. Concurrent IV. % Interviewed V. Blind Interviews RCE Level of Evidence
Gaynes 2010[12] M-3	MINI	I. Not reported (eligible patients were age 18 or older, English speaking, mentally competent, and attending primary care academic family medicine clinic) II. 54% of those approached (n=723)	I. Mean age = 45 years 71% female 67% white, 28% black, 5% other 49% married 55% high school education or less 21% unemployed II. complete date for 89% (647/723 who consented	I. One family medicine clinic, sample similar to overall clinic II. Fair (In person or telephone, research assistant) III. Yes, within 30 days IV. 89% V. Yes **Level of Evidence: I**
Houston 2011[50] PDT-4A	SCID	I. Not reported (eligible patients were age 18 or older, non-psychotic, and seen in primary care clinic) Not reported, 343 of those who completed an initial questionnaire were "qualified" for the study after initial interview by investigating physician	I. Mean age = 47 years 69% female 86% white 48% married II. 78% (343/440)	I. One primary care clinic II. Fair (telephone, "trained rater") III. Not reported IV. Not reported V. Not reported **Level of Evidence: IV**
Means-Christensen 2006[51] ADD	CIDI	I. Not reported II. 61% of patients approached (7738/12724)	I. Mean age = 42 years 62% female 65% Caucasian, 16% African American, 10% Hispanic, 4% Asian, 5% other II. 867 of 1494 that screened positive (58%) agreed to interview; 569 (38%) completed interview 452 of random sample of 1107 that screened negative (41%) agreed to interview; 232 (21%) completed interview	I. More interviews among positive screens II. Fair (telephone, trained CIDI interviewers) III. Yes, median of 14 days IV. 38% of those that screened positive; 21% of random sample of those that screened negative V. No **Level of Evidence: IV**
Kroenke 2007[14] GAD	SCID	I. Not reported II. 92% (2740/2982) completed questionnaire (including GAD-7); of 2740, the first 2149 were used for development and validation of the GAD-7	I. Mean age=47years 69% female 81% non-Hispanic white, 7% black, 9% Hispanic, 3% other 65% married 34% high school education or less II. 77% (1654/2149) agreed to interview; 58% (965/1654) randomly selected for interview	I. Yes-15 primary care sites in 12 states (part of research network) II. Fair (telephone, 1 of 2 mental health professionals) III. Yes, approximately 1 week IV. 100% (this analysis based on those who completed GAD-7 and were interviewed) V. Yes **Level of Evidence: I**

QUADAS = QUality Assessment of Studies of Diagnostic Accuracy included in Systematic reviews tool (Whiting 2003)[6]
RCE = Rational Clinical Examination (Simel 2008)[7] (see Appendix C)
*Baseline data from n=188 (56% of those who completed an initial screen)

APPENDIX F. SPECIFIC ASSOCIATION OF RCE LEVEL OF EVIDENCE RATINGS TO QUADAS ITEM RATINGS AS APPLIED IN THIS REVIEW

RCE Level of Evidence Rating	QUADAS Item 1 Sample size of screening sample	QUADAS Item 2 Representativeness of screening sample viz. target population/ selection method	QUADAS Item 3 Sample size/ representativeness of Interview sample viz. screening sample	QUADAS Item 4 Quality of gold standard and its administration	QUADAS Item 5 Blinded/concurrent diagnostic evaluations
I	Large	Representative of target population/randomly selected or consecutive sample	All of screening sample or randomly selected representative sample	In person by trained diagnostician	Yes
II	Small	Representative of target population/randomly selected or consecutive sample	All of screening sample or randomly selected representative sample	In person by trained diagnostician	Yes
III*	Small or Large	Representative sample or convenience/non-representative sample	Random selection or non-representative interview sample	In person or by telephone by trained diagnostician	Yes
IV†	Small	Convenience/non-representative sample	Non-random interview sample	Telephone by trained research assistants	No
V			*Not included in Systematic Review*		

QUADAS = QUality Assessment of Studies of Diagnostic Accuracy included in Systematic reviews tool (Whiting 2003)[6]

RCE = Rational Clinical Examination (Simel 2008)[7] (see Appendix C)

*Level III studies have either a small sample size and lower ratings on QUADAS 2 or QUADAS 3, or a larger sample size and lower ratings on both QUADAS 2 and QUADAS 3

†Level IV studies may have a higher rating on one of the QUADAS 1-4 criteria but have lower ratings in the other 3 criteria